Pediatric Occupational Therapy

HANDBOOK

A Guide to Diagnoses and Evidence-Based Interventions

PATRICIA BOWYER • **SUSAN M. CAHILL**

EdD, OTR/L, BCN

Associate Professor and Associate
  Director
Texas Woman's University at
  Houston
The Texas Medical Center
Houston, Texas

MAEA, OTR/L

Clinical Assistant Professor
Department of Occupational
  Therapy
University of Illinois at Chicago
Chicago, Illinois

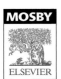

MOSBY

ELSEVIER

11830 Westline Industrial Drive
St. Louis, Missouri 63146

PEDIATRIC OCCUPATIONAL THERAPY HANDBOOK:
A GUIDE TO DIAGNOSES AND EVIDENCE-BASED
INTERVENTIONS
Copyright © 2009 by Mosby, Inc., an affiliate of Elsevier Inc.

ISBN: 978-0-323-05341-9

Notice

Library of Congress Cataloging in Publication Data
Bowyer, Patricia.
  Pediatric occupational therapy handbook : a guide to diagnoses and evidence-based interventions
/ Patricia Bowyer, Susan M. Cahill.—1st ed.
    p. ; cm.
  Includes bibliographical references and index.
  ISBN 978-0-323-05341-9 (pbk. : alk. paper) 1. Occupational therapy for children—Handbooks,
manuals, etc. I. Cahill, Susan M. II. Title.
  [DNLM: 1. Occupational Therapy—Handbooks. 2. Child. 3. Developmental Disabilities—
diagnosis—Handbooks. 4. Disabled Children—rehabilitation—Handbooks. 5. Evidence-Based
Medicine—methods—Handbooks. WS 39 B788p 2009]
  RJ53.O25B69 2009
  615.8'515083—dc22

                                                                                          2008018946

Vice President and Publisher: Linda Duncan
Senior Editor: Kathy Falk
Senior Developmental Editor: Melissa Kuster Deutsch
Editorial Assistant: Lindsay Westbrook
Publishing Services Manager: Patricia Tannian
Project Manager: John Casey
Design Manager: Amy Buxton

Working together to grow
libraries in developing countries
www.elsevier.com | www.bookaid.org | www.sabre.org

ELSEVIER   BOOK AID International   Sabre Foundation

Printed in United States of America

Last digit is the print number: 9 8 7 6 5 4 3 2 1

To those who will benefit from the information contained within—students, practitioners, children and their families.

And to Bobby and Brian, who live in the moment, know what is important, and help dreams come true.

Preface

Pediatric Occupational Therapy Handbook: A Guide to Diagnoses and Evidence-Based Interventions is designed to provide occupational therapy students and practitioners with an easily accessible reference for common diagnoses found in pediatric practice. Students and clinicians currently refer to multiple sources to gather such information, as well as attempt to carry and store numerous large textbooks to use as a reference when in need of information. *Pediatric Occupational Therapy Handbook* consolidates all of the essential information into a single handy reference, eliminating the cumbersome task of leafing through multiple books.

Organization

The manual is organized alphabetically by diagnosis. Information in each section reflects the occupational therapy practice framework, as well as policies governing the various areas of pediatric practice, such as community settings, early intervention services, school systems practice, and clinic-based services.

Who Will Benefit From This Book?

This guide provides occupational therapy practitioners and students working in busy clinical settings with a compact, accessible, A-Z evidence-based resource on a multitude of pediatric conditions. Because the essential information is consolidated into this handy reference, the need to search through multiple resources is eliminated. The information is based on current research and thus provides the information and detail necessary for making sound decisions during clinical intervention.

Distinctive Features

The handbook includes a consistent formatting for each pediatric disease:

- Epidemiology
- Impact on performance skills and client factors
- Precautions
- Suggested assessment tools
- Intervention strategies
- Case examples
- Web resources
- Recommendations for further reading

Acknowledgments

This book is the result of recognizing a need that we observed in the classroom and in various pediatric practice settings. The pages of this book will hopefully be a place where students and practitioners can begin the process of implementing evidence-based practice. As with any endeavor of this nature, there are many who help an idea become a reality. We would like to thank the Elsevier team who supported us from beginning to end in making the idea of this book come to life: Kathy Falk, Melissa Kuster, John Casey, and Tara Knittel. Your guidance and assistance made it possible. We would also like to thank our families and mentors. You continually inspire us to seek new challenges and do great things.

Patricia Bowyer
Susan M. Cahill

Contents

Section I *Guide to Pediatric Practice*

1 Using the Occupational Therapy Practice Framework in Pediatric Practice, *3*
2 Using Evidence to Guide Occupational Therapy Practice, *9*

Section II *Guide to Diagnoses and Interventions*

3 Achondroplasia, *17*
4 Acquired Brain Injury, *21*
5 Acquired Immunodeficiency Syndrome, *25*
6 Albers-Schönberg Disease, *29*
7 Amblyopia, *33*
8 Anemia, *37*
9 Angelman Syndrome, *41*
10 Anorexia, *45*
11 Anxiety, *49*
12 Apnea, *53*
13 Arthrogryposis Multiplex Congenita, *57*
14 Asthma, *63*
15 Attention Deficit/Hyperactivity Disorder, *67*
16 Autism Spectrum Disorders, *73*
17 Bipolar Disorder, *81*
18 Brachial Plexus Injury, *85*
19 Bronchopulmonary Dysplasia, *89*
20 Bulimia, *93*
21 Cerebral Palsy, *97*
22 Cleft Palate, *107*
23 Conduct Disorder, *111*
24 Congenital Clubfoot (*Talipes Equinovarus*), *115*
25 Congenital Heart Defects, *119*

26 Congenital Obstructive Hydrocephalus, *123*
27 Cri du Chat Syndrome, *127*
28 Cystic Fibrosis, *131*
29 Depression, *135*
30 Developmental Coordination Disorder, *139*
31 Disseminated Intravascular Coagulation, *143*
32 Down Syndrome (Trisomy 21), *145*
33 Dysrhythmias, *151*
34 Edwards' syndrome (Trisomy 18), *153*
35 Epilepsy (Seizure Disorder), *157*
36 Fetal Alcohol Syndrome Disorders, *161*
37 Fragile X Syndrome, *165*
38 Galactosemia, *169*
39 Gastroschisis, *173*
40 Hemophilia, *175*
41 Hydrocephalus, *179*
42 Hyperbilirubinemia, *185*
43 Hypoxic-Ischemic Encephalopathy, *187*
44 Intellectual Disabilities, *191*
45 Intraventricular Hemorrhage, *195*
46 Juvenile Diabetes, *199*
47 Juvenile Rheumatoid Arthritis, *201*
48 Klinefelter's Syndrome, *205*
49 Learning Disabilities, *207*
50 Legg-Calvé-Perthes Disease, *213*
51 Lesch-Nyhan Syndrome, *217*
52 Lordosis, *221*
53 Marfan Syndrome, *225*
54 Meconium Aspiration Syndrome, *229*
55 Micrognathia, *233*
56 Mononucleosis, *237*
57 Muscular Dystrophy, *241*
58 Necrotizing Enterocolitis, *247*
59 Neonatal Respiratory Distress Syndrome, *251*
60 Neurofibromatosis, *255*
61 Nystagmus, *261*
62 Obesity, *265*

63 Oppositional Defiant Disorder, *269*
64 Osteogenesis Imperfecta, *273*
65 Patau's Syndrome (Trisomy 13), *277*
66 Periventricular Leukomalacia, *283*
67 Persistent Pulmonary Hypertension, *287*
68 Phenylketonuria, *291*
69 Pica, *295*
70 Posttraumatic Stress Disorder, *299*
71 Pneumonia, *303*
72 Prader-Willi Syndrome, *307*
73 Retinopathy of Prematurity, *313*
74 Rheumatic Heart Disease, *317*
75 Scoliosis, *321*
76 Separation Anxiety and Social Phobia, *327*
77 Sensory Processing Disorder, *331*
78 Sepsis, *335*
79 Sickle Cell Anemia, *339*
80 Spina Bifida, *343*
81 Spinal Muscular Atrophy, *347*
82 Strabismus, *351*
83 Tay-Sachs Disease, *355*
84 Tourette Syndrome, *361*

Appendices

A Websites for Research, *367*
B Assessment Tools, *371*

Guide to Pediatric Practice

1

❖

Using the Occupational Therapy Practice Framework in Pediatric Practice

Pediatric occupational therapists deliver services day in and day out. Whether speaking with a parent, a teacher, a physician, or another professional, many occupational therapists find themselves in daily interactions that require the use of a common language. As members of the occupational therapy profession, we uphold a common belief system that values occupation as both a means and an outcome for our young clients. The commonalities that exist and the beliefs we share are what make up our profession (Kielhofner, 2004).

Creation of a Unified Language

The profession of occupational therapy has grown and changed since its beginnings almost 100 years ago. Because of the changes within the profession as well as in the provision of occupational therapy services, there has been a need to provide a structure that helps to organize knowledge and the language that guides practice; helps unite practitioners, educators, and researchers; and communicates the profession's focus on occupation and daily activities to individuals outside the profession.

The American Occupational Therapy Association (AOTA) has tried to facilitate the use of common language among occupational therapy practitioners and to improve the general public's understanding of the services we provide. The result of the initial effort, the Uniform Terminology (AOTA, 1994), has evolved into the Occupational Therapy Practice Framework (OTPF or the Framework) (AOTA, 2002).

Occupational Therapy Practice Framework

The Framework begins with an explanation of the profession's domain. Figure 1-1 shows the domains of practice. Understanding the domains of occupational therapy practice is important because it helps to frame our areas of assessment and intervention. In Figure 1-1 the domains that are addressed through occupational therapy are organized under an overarching concern of practitioners, namely, engagement in occupation to support participation in meaningful contexts. Occupational engagement in meaningful contexts is then broken down into more specific areas, which include performance areas of occupation, performance skills, performance patterns, context, activity demands, and client factors.

The next key component of the Framework is used to direct the service delivery of occupational therapy in all practice settings, including pediatrics. The Framework is organized into three categories: evaluation, intervention, and outcomes (engagement in occupation to support participation). Box 1-1 and Figure 1-2 provide an overview of the Framework.

The first area is evaluation (see Box 1-1). Evaluation is described as the occupational profile and analysis of performance. The next area is intervention. This includes the intervention plan, intervention implementation, and intervention review. Last is the outcomes process. Outcomes are the results of the intervention process. Assessment of outcomes is when the practitioner determines how well OT intervention

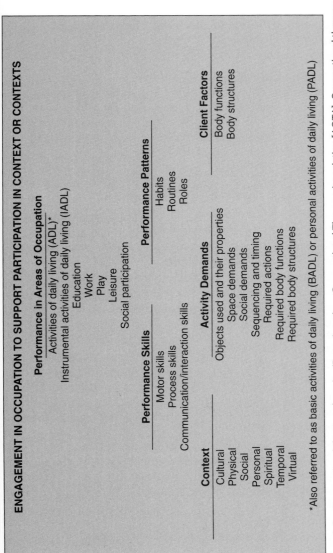

Figure 1-1 Occupational therapy domain. (From American Occupational Therapy Association [AOTA]: Occupational therapy practice framework: domain and process, *Am J Occup Ther* 56:611, 2002.)

BOX 1-1
Framework Process of Service Delivery as Applied within the Profession's Domain

Evaluation

Occupational Profile

The initial step in the evaluation process that provides an understanding of the client's occupational history and experiences, patterns of daily living, interests, values, and needs. The client's problems and concerns about performing occupations and daily life activities are identified, and the client's priorities are determined.

Analysis of Occupational Performance

The step in the evaluation process during which the client's assets, problems, or potential problems are more specifically identified. Actual performance is often observed in context to identify what supports performance and what hinders performance. Performance skills, performance patterns, context(s), activity demands, and client factors are all considered, but only selected aspects may be specifically assessed. Targeted outcomes are identified.

Intervention

Intervention Plan

A plan that will guide actions taken and that is developed in collaboration with the client. It is based on selected theories, frames of reference, and evidence. Outcomes to be targeted are confirmed.

Intervention Implementation

Ongoing actions taken to influence and support improved client performance. Interventions are directed at identified outcomes. Client's response is monitored and documented.

Intervention Review

A review of the implementation plan and process as well as its progress toward targeted outcomes.

BOX 1-1

Framework Process of Service Delivery as Applied within the Profession's Domain—cont'd

> ***Outcomes (Engagement in Occupation to Support Participation)***
>
> Outcomes
>
> Determination of success in reaching desired targeted outcomes. Outcome assessment information is used to plan future actions with the client and to evaluate the service program (i.e., program evaluation).

From American Occupational Therapy Association (AOTA): Occupational Therapy Practice Framework: domain and process, *Am J Occup Ther* 56:614, 2002.

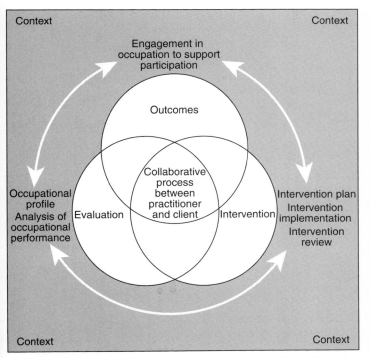

Figure 1-2 Framework collaborative process model. Illustration of the Framework emphasizing client-practitioner interactive relationship and interactive nature of the service delivery process. (From American Occupational Therapy Association [AOTA]: Occupational therapy practice framework: domain and process, *Am J Occup Ther* 56:614, 2002.)

addressed the ability of the clients to engage in occupations that support participation in their own lives.

Figure 1-2 shows how all the areas interact and are related, as well as how the relationship between the therapist and client is central to the process. The emphasis in practice is the relationship between you, the therapist, and your client, as affected by the service delivery process.

REFERENCES

American Occupational Therapy Association (AOTA): Uniform terminology for occupational therapy, third edition, *Am J Occup Ther* 48:1047, 1994.

American Occupational Therapy Association (AOTA): Occupational therapy practice framework: domain and process, *Am J Occup Ther* 56:609, 2002.

Kielhofner G: *Conceptual foundations of occupational therapy, ed 3*, Philadelphia, 2004, FA Davis.

2

❖

Using Evidence to Guide Occupational Therapy Practice

Occupational therapists providing services to children and their families are becoming increasingly aware of the need for evidence-based practice. In addition to the knowledge and evidence they have gained from experience, pediatric practitioners are being asked to use other sources of information to guide their clinical decision-making processes.

The notion of engaging in evidence-based practice can be daunting to many. Sometimes there is confusion over where to begin. This chapter outlines the steps a practitioner can follow in creating an evidence-based practice.

Step 1: Form the Question

Many occupational therapists engaging in evidence-based practice start by forming a clinical question to guide their research. Often the question will be aimed at uncovering valuable information that supports best practices with a particular child or client. At other times the question will be geared toward increasing overall knowledge and skills of the occupational therapist. Examples of clinical questions that lead to evidence-based inquiry include the following:

- What occupational performance issues may be of concern to a child and his or her family?
- Which assessment tool has been found to be both valid and reliable for children of a given age or to measure a specific skill or theoretic construct?
- What potential impact might a specific medical condition have on the occupational performance of a child at home, at school, and/or in the community?
- Which intervention techniques or strategies have been found to be the most effective?
- What are the recommendations and contraindications for using a specific intervention technique or strategy?
- Has this intervention technique or strategy been effective in supporting the occupational performance of this child?

Step 2: Uncover the Best Evidence

Your clinical question, as well as your experience using various resources, will likely guide the approach you use to search for evidence. The ease and accessibility of the Internet often make it the first place occupational therapists turn to for new information. Despite the wealth of information that is available, not all websites are created equally.

Occupational Therapy Search Engines

Many national and local occupational therapy associations provide members with access to their online publications archives. In addition, several search engines are dedicated to providing occupational therapists with current information to guide evidence-based practice. Starting your search with an occupational therapy organization or search engine will likely yield positive results.

OT Seeker (www.otseeker.com) was developed by faculty from two universities in Australia. It is a free database that will allow you to search using keywords to find abstracts related to your clinical question. The administrators at OT Seeker have appraised each study and provide a rating to help therapists interpret the validity of the findings. OT Seeker also provides an expansive list of other websites to investigate, including those that provide "how to" checklists that outline the appraisal process.

OT-CATS (www.otcats.com) was also developed in Australia and provides occupational therapists with access to evidence summaries related to many clinical topics of interest. The site also includes a template that is a helpful guide for those who wish to complete their own review of a topic or summarize information related to a clinical question.

Other Scholarly Search Engines

Recent graduates and students doing fieldwork may feel limited by not having access to the resources they grew accustomed to using in school, because many institutions of higher education restrict access to their electronic journals. Despite this challenge, several avenues can be explored when trying to search for the best evidence to guide occupational therapy.

First, many public libraries subscribe to electronic databases, which makes accessing electronic journals easy. If the database does not have the journal you are seeking, chat with the librarian and inquire about other possible means for accessing this information. Some libraries share resources through an interlibrary loan agreement, which means you might have access to more than you think.

Another possible solution is to contact a local community college or other institution of higher education. Some provide the opportunity to purchase a library pass for a nominal fee to use over the course of an academic quarter or semester. Often this pass will give you access to electronic databases, as well as other resources such as books and videos.

Finally, you might also try searching the National Institute of Health's free online digital archive, PubMed (www. pubmedcentral.nih.gov). PubMed provides anyone with Internet capability with an abundance of free information and is an excellent place to visit on a regular basis.

Popular Search Engines and Websites

Using keywords to locate information through popular search engines often produces voluminous results that require a great deal of time to look through and evaluate. It will take you some time to figure out which sites are worthwhile to come back to and which are not.

If you are exploring online, consider starting with sites that are recognized as having a good reputation. Many national foundations and organizations provide valuable information, as do many institutions of higher education, governmental bodies, and clearinghouses. In addition, publishers of commercially available assessments often provide a list of references or other information related to the psychometric properties of these tools and how they were developed.

Other Sources of Information

In your search for evidence to support your practice, you might also choose to explore other sources, such as continuing education courses and Web-based discussion boards. Both provide good opportunities for networking with other occupational therapists as well as avenues for discussion of clinical questions and sharing of therapy outcomes.

Step 3: Evaluate the Information and Determine How It Can Be Applied in Your Practice

Once you have collected information related to your question, it is important to evaluate it. Research articles from peer-reviewed journals will provide you with better evidence than informational websites geared toward the general public.

When you start examining the articles you have collected, it is important to do so in a reflective and objective manner. For example, you may discover findings related to a certain intervention that suggest it is not effective. If you are

TABLE 2-1
Hierarchy of Levels of Evidence for Evidence-Based Practice

Level	Description
I	Strong evidence from at least one systematic review of multiple well-designed randomized controlled trials
II	Strong evidence from at least one properly designed randomized controlled trial of appropriate size
III	Evidence from well-designed trials without randomization, single group before and after, cohort, time series, or matched case-controlled studies
IV	Evidence from well-designed nonexperimental studies from more than one center or research group
V	Opinions of respected authorities, based on clinical evidence, descriptive studies, or reports of expert committees

From Moore A, McQuay H, Gray J: Evidence-based everything, *Bandolier* 1:1, 1995.

comfortable using tools to assist you in evaluating the level of the evidence, you can confidently apply what you have learned to your practice.

Established hierarchies can be used to rank the level of evidence found in published research studies (Table 2-1). However, if you are unfamiliar with reading research articles, this can be a time-consuming and cumbersome task and you might consider learning more about using evidence to make clinical decisions. The American Occupational Therapy Foundation (www.aotf.org) provides resources for completing a self-study related to evidence-based practice that many clinicians find extremely helpful.

Appendix A includes a listing and description of some websites you can use to start your search.

FURTHER READING

Berg C, LaVesser P: Incorporating evidence into practice, *Dev Disabil Spec Interest Sect Q* 28:1, 2005.

Collins A: Using evidence to guide decision making in the educational setting, *School Syst Spec Interest Sect Q* 13:1, 2006.

Dysart A, Tomlin G: Factors related to evidence-based practice among U.S. occupational therapy clinicians, *Am J Occup Ther* 56:275, 2002.

Holm M: Eleanor Clarke Slagle lecture—our mandate for the new millennium: evidence-based practice, *Am J Occup Ther* 54:575, 2000.

Law M, Pollock N, Stewart D: Evidence-based occupational therapy: concepts and strategies, *N Z J Occup Ther* 51:14, 2004.

McCluskey A, Cusik A: Strategies for introducing evidence-based practice and changing clinician behaviour: a manager's toolbox, *Aust Occup Ther J* 49:63, 2002.

Moore A, McQuay H, Gray J: Evidence-based everything, *Bandolier* 1:1, 1995.

Ottenbacher K, Tickle-Degnen L, Hasselkus B: Therapists awake! The challenge of evidence-based occupational therapy, *Am J Occup Ther* 56:247, 2002.

Sackett D, Rosenberg W, Gray J, et al: Evidence-based medicine: what it is and what it isn't, *BMJ* 312:71, 1996.

Sarracino T: Using evidence to inform school-based practice, *School Syst Spec Interest Sect Q* 9:1, 2002.

Tickle-Degnen L: Evidence-based practice forum—communicating with clients, family members, and colleagues about research evidence, *Am J Occup Ther* 54:341, 2000.

Tickle-Degnen L: Evidence-based practice forum—gathering current research evidence to enhance clinical reasoning, *Am J Occup Ther* 54:102, 2000.

Tickle-Degnen L: Evidence-based practice forum—monitoring and documenting evidence during assessment and intervention, *Am J Occup Ther* 54:434, 2000.

Tickle-Degnen L: Evidence-based practice forum—organizing, evaluating, and using evidence in occupational therapy practice, *Am J Occup Ther* 53:537, 1999.

Tickle-Degnen L: Evidence-based practice forum—what is the best evidence to use in practice? *Am J Occup Ther* 54:218, 2000.

Guide to Diagnoses and Interventions

Information presented in this section is formatted to match the Occupational Therapy Practice Framework. Each chapter includes the following:

- Epidemiology
- Impact on Performance Skills
- Impact on Client Factors (Body Functions and Structures)
- Precautions
    - Impact on Performance Skills
    - Impact on Client Factors (Body Functions and Structures)
- Evaluation (including specific assessment tools, methods for data collection)
    - Clinical observations
    - Interviews with child and family
    - Assessment tools
- Suggested Assessment Tools*
- Interventions
- Case Example
- Web Resources
- Further Reading

*The lists are suggestions for evaluation tools but do not include exhaustive lists. Descriptions of the assessments are found in Appendix B.

3

❖

Achondroplasia

A

Epidemiology

Achondroplasia, also referred to as *dwarfism,* is a genetic disorder that affects one in every 15,000 to 40,000 births. It is caused by a genetic mutation of the fibroblast growth factor receptor gene 3 (FGFR3).

Impact on Performance Skills

Children with achondroplasia may demonstrate delays in motor skills such as the following:
- Posture
- Mobility
- Coordination
- Strength

   Typically, children with achondroplasia will not demonstrate delays in process or communication and interaction skills.

Impact on Client Factors (Body Functions and Structures)

The mutation of the FGFR3 gene results in abnormal cartilage development and shortened bones.

   Individuals with achondroplasia are often short in stature, typically not growing taller than 52 inches in adulthood, and have shortened limbs. In addition, they have short fingers and toes, as well as lower extremity deformations such as

17

A

varus (they are bowlegged) or valgus (they are knock-kneed). Additional features of individuals with achondroplasia include low tone, a large head, and a high forehead.

Precautions

Impact on Performance Skills

Some children with achondroplasia experience hydrocephalus and may have a ventricular shunt. Signs of shunt dysfunction include changes in the child's communication and interaction skills, changes in process skills, complaints of headache, and signs of fever.

Impact on Client Factors (Body Functions and Structures)

Children with achondroplasia are at risk for developing kyphosis, and adults with achondroplasia are at risk for developing lordosis and spinal stenosis.

Individuals with achondroplasia are at risk for obesity.

Evaluation

- Checklists or observations related to home, school, and community accessibility or child-environment fit
- Clinical observations
- Interviews with child and family
- Assessment tools

Suggested Assessment Tools

- Canadian Occupational Performance Measure (COPM)
- Child Occupational Self Assessment (COSA)
- Children's Assessment of Participation and Enjoyment (CAPE)
- Pediatric Evaluation of Disability Inventory (PEDI)
- Pediatric Interest Profile (PIP)
- School Function Assessment (SFA)
- School Setting Interview (SSI)
- Short Child Occupational Profile (SCOPE)

INTERVENTIONS

A

- Environmental accommodations and modifications
- Task accommodations and modifications
- Joint protection to reduce likelihood of deformity and subsequent pain
- Positioning in high chairs, strollers, and other types of seating that provide adequate back support and decrease risk of deformity
- Interest exploration for physically active leisure participation

Case Example

James is a 14-year-old boy with achondroplasia who will be transitioning to high school next year. Before his transition meeting, James visits the high school with his occupational therapist to determine what environmental and task modifications may be necessary to ensure that he has full access to all areas of the school and the curricular materials. ❖

WEB RESOURCES

Little People of America
www.lpaonline.org

March of Dimes
www.marchofdimes.com

FURTHER READING

Carter E, Davis J, Raggio C: Advances in understanding etiology of achondroplasia and review of management, *Curr Opin Pediatr* 19:32, 2007.

4

❖

Acquired Brain Injury

Epidemiology

Acquired brain injury (ABI) is an insult to the brain that occurs at or after birth. ABIs may be a result of injury or trauma to the head, anoxia, infections, neurologic incidents, or tumors. Most ABIs are preventable; however, ABI is recognized as a leading cause of death to children and young adults in the United States.

Impact on Performance Skills

Children with ABI may experience difficulty in various motor, process and communication, and interaction skills depending on the areas of the brain that were affected by the injury.

Performance skills affected may include the following:
- Posture
- Mobility
- Coordination
- Strength and effort
- Energy
- Knowledge
- Temporal organization
- Organizing space and objects
- Adaptation
- Physicality
- Information exchange
- Relations

Performance patterns, such as habits, roles, and routines, may also be affected by ABI.

Impact on Client Factors (Body Functions and Structures)

Injury to the brain may result in changes to the following client factors:

- Mental functions
- Sensory functions
- Movement-related functions
- Respiratory functions
- Voice and speech functions

Precautions

Children with ABI may have seizures, as well as decreased safety awareness and increased incidence of impulsivity. In addition, children with ABI may have a ventricular shunt due to hydrocephalus.

Signs of shunt dysfunction include the following:

- Changes in the child's communication and interaction skills
- Changes in process skills
- Complaints of headache and signs of fever

Children with ABI are more at risk for depression, irritability, and anxiety.

Evaluation

- Clinical observations
- Interviews with child and family
- Assessment tools

Suggested Assessment Tools

- Assessment of Motor and Process Skills (AMPS)
- Árnadóttir OT-ADL Neurobehavioral Evaluation (A-ONE)
- Behavioral Assessment of the Dysexecutive Syndrome (BADS)
- Canadian Occupational Performance Measure (COPM)

- Child and Adolescent Social Perception Measure
- Child Occupational Self Assessment (COSA)
- Children's Assessment of Participation and Enjoyment (CAPE)
- Dynamic Occupational Therapy Cognitive Assessment for Children (DOTCA-Ch)
- Lowenstein Occupational Therapy Cognitive Assessment (LOTCA)
- Mayo-Portland Adaptability Inventory (MPAI)
- Miller Function and Participation Scales (M-FUN-S)
- Pediatric Evaluation of Disability Inventory (PEDI)
- Pediatric Interest Profile (PIP)
- Pediatric Volitional Questionnaire (PVQ)
- Perceived Efficacy and Goal Setting System (PEGS)
- School Assessment of Motor and Process Skills (School AMPS)
- School Function Assessment (SFA)
- School Setting Interview (SSI)
- Short Child Occupational Profile (SCOPE)
- Social Skills Rating System
- Test of Everyday Attention for Children (TEA-Ch)
- WeeFIM

INTERVENTIONS

- Activities of daily living (ADL) or instrumental activities of daily living (IADL) retraining
- Environmental accommodations and modifications
- Task accommodations and modifications
- Interventions to increase posture, mobility, coordination, strength, and effort
- Tone management
- Interventions to increase safety awareness, knowledge, temporal organization, organizing space and objects, adaptation, physicality, and information exchange
- Social skills retraining
- Caregiver and family coaching

A

Case Example

Sarah is a 4-year-old child with ABI status after a motor vehicle accident. Sarah presents with increased tone in her right upper and lower extremities. She wears an ankle-foot orthosis (AFO) but walks without assistance. Sarah is right-dominant and before her car accident was independent in feeding and age-appropriate self-care. The occupational therapist is working with Sarah to help her regain functional independence in meaningful activities while addressing her motor, process, and communication and interaction skills. ❖

WEB RESOURCES

Brain Injury Association of America
www.biausa.org

Educating Educators About ABI
www.abieducation.com

FURTHER READING

Hawley C, Ward A, Magnay A, Long J: Outcomes following childhood head injury: a population study, *J Neurol Neurosurg Psychiatr* 75:737, 2004.

Kieslich M, Marquardt G, Galow G, et al: Neurological and mental outcome after severe head injury in childhood: a long-term follow-up of 318 children, *Disabil Rehabil* 23:665, 2001.

5

❖

Acquired Immunodeficiency Syndrome

Epidemiology

Acquired immunodeficiency syndrome (AIDS) is caused by damage to the immune system after infection with human immunodeficiency virus (HIV). AIDS involves the diminished function of the immune system and a CD4 cell count below 200 cells/mm^3 or the presence of at least one opportunistic infection in an individual who is HIV positive.

There are approximately 5500 reported cases of children living with HIV or AIDS in the United States.

Medical treatment for individuals living with HIV or AIDS has greatly improved over the last 10 years, and many children with HIV or AIDS will not experience occupational performance issues related to this condition.

Impact on Performance Skills

If AIDS advances or children contract opportunistic infections, they may grow to experience difficulty with motor, process, and communication and interaction skills.

Impact on Client Factors (Body Functions and Structures)

• Immunologic systems functions

Precautions

A

Owing to their compromised immune systems, children with AIDS are at higher risk for contracting opportunistic infections such as the following:

- *Pneumocystis carinii* pneumonia (PCP)
- *Candida* (thrush)
- Herpes simplex virus (HSV)
- *Mycobacterium avium* complex (MAC)
- *Cryptosporidium*
- Cytomegalovirus (CMV)
- *Cryptococcus*
- Toxoplasmosis
- Herpes zoster
- Tuberculosis
- Chicken pox

Evaluation

- Clinical observations
- Interviews with child and family
- Assessment tools

Suggested Assessment Tools

- Alberta Infant Motor Scale (AIMS)
- Bayley Scale of Infant Development (BSID)
- Canadian Occupational Performance Measure (COPM)
- Child Occupational Self Assessment (COSA)
- Children's Assessment of Participation and Enjoyment (CAPE)
- Coping Inventory
- Denver Developmental Screening Test (DDST)
- Hawaii Early Learning Profile (HELP)
- Miller Function and Participation Scales (M-FUN-S)
- Peabody Developmental Motor Scales 2, Revised (PDMS-2)
- Pediatric Evaluation of Disability Inventory (PEDI)
- Pediatric Interest Profile (PIP)
- Pediatric Volitional Questionnaire (PVQ)
- School Function Assessment (SFA)

- School Setting Interview (SSI)
- Short Child Occupational Profile (SCOPE)
- WeeFIM

A

INTERVENTIONS

- Support for the development of habits and routines related to health maintenance and medication management
- Advocacy and self-determination skill development
- Accommodations and modification in educational and community settings
- Intervention in areas of occupational performance
- Prevocational skill
- Volitional development

Case Example

The occupational therapist leads a group on medical rights for a group of teenagers in the community who are HIV positive. Individuals who participate in the group learn how to navigate the public medical system and advocate for their needs. ❖

WEB RESOURCES

Elizabeth Glaser Pediatric AIDS Foundation
www.pedaids.org

AIDS Alliance for Children, Youth, and Families
www.aids-alliance.org/aids_alliance/index.html

FURTHER READING

Brady M: Treatment of human immunodeficiency virus infection and its associated complications in children, *J Clin Pharmacol* 34:17, 1994.

6

❖

Albers-Schönberg Disease

Epidemiology

Albers-Schönberg disease is also known as *osteopetrosis* and *marble-bone disease.* It is a rare genetic condition that affects bone formation. Albers-Schönberg disease is present in one of every 20,000 to 500,000 births. Children with this condition are typically diagnosed through x-ray examinations and bone density tests. Compression of cranial nerves is a complication of Albers-Schönberg disease and may lead to blindness and deafness. In addition, children with this condition may experience cerebral vascular accidents and hematologic difficulties.

Two types of Albers-Schönberg disease affect children: infantile and intermediate. Infantile Albers-Schönberg disease is typically diagnosed shortly after birth. The intermediate type is usually diagnosed before the child turns 10 years old. Both types are treated medically with bone marrow transplants and vitamin D supplements.

Impact on Performance Skills

- Posture
- Mobility
- Coordination

- Strength and effort
- Energy

Impact on Client Factors (Body Functions and Structures)
- Movement-related functions

Precautions
Before undergoing bone marrow transplants, children with Albers-Schönberg disease are at high risk for fractures owing to the limited stress their bones can support. They are also at high risk for infection and may have poor dentition, which may affect feeding.

Evaluation
- Clinical observations
- Interviews with child and family
- Assessment tools

Suggested Assessment Tools
- Alberta Infant Motor Scale (AIMS)
- Bayley Scale of Infant Development (BSID)
- Canadian Occupational Performance Measure (COPM)
- Children's Assessment of Participation and Enjoyment (CAPE)
- Denver Developmental Screening Test (DDST)
- Hawaii Early Learning Profile (HELP)
- Miller Function and Participation Scales (M-FUN-S)
- Peabody Developmental Motor Scales 2, Revised (PDMS-2)
- Pediatric Evaluation of Disability Inventory (PEDI)
- School Function Assessment (SFA)
- School Setting Interview (SSI)
- Short Child Occupational Profile (SCOPE)
- Toddler and Infant Motor Evaluation (TIME)
- WeeFIM

INTERVENTIONS

- Interventions to support the development of posture, mobility, coordination, strength, and effort
- Support for participation in self-care and play
- Environmental accommodations and modifications, including those related to hearing and vision loss
- Task accommodations and modifications, including those related to hearing and vision loss
- Caregiver and family coaching
- Consultation and intervention related to proper nutrition and feeding

Case Example

Jose is a 3-year-old child with Albers-Schönberg disease and blindness. He is having difficulty with eating because of poorly formed and decaying teeth. Jose will not eat protein-rich foods, such as beef and chicken, because they are difficult for him to chew. In addition, his mother continues to feed him because she thinks self-feeding would be too difficult owing to Jose's vision impairment. The occupational therapist consults with Jose's mother and a nutritionist regarding protein-rich alternatives to meet Jose's dietary needs, as well as the manner in which these foods could be presented to him to encourage self-feeding. ❖

WEB RESOURCES

Osteopetrosis Support Trust
www.osteopetrosis.co.uk

Information about osteopetrosis from the American Academy of Physicians
www.aafp.org/afp/980315ap/carolino.html

FURTHER READING

Charles J, Key L: Developmental spectrum of children with congenital osteopetrosis, *J Pediatr* 132:371, 1998.

7

❖

Amblyopia

Epidemiology

Amblyopia, also called "*lazy eye*," is a result of a misalignment or muscle imbalance of a child's eye and affects the child's ability to use both eyes together. One eye gets stronger while the one with amblyopia progressively becomes weaker. If the condition is left untreated, vision loss can occur in the amblyopic eye. Signs and symptoms of amblyopia include difficulty with depth perception and visible turning in or out of one eye. It is estimated that 3% to 5% of children will experience amblyopia.

Patching is a common medical treatment used to treat amblyopia. Physicians may alternately prescribe eye drops to blur the vision of the unaffected eye and avoid patching. In addition, other vision conditions, which are sometimes the cause of amblyopia, will be treated simultaneously.

Impact on Performance Skills
- Organizing space and objects
  - Searches and locates
  - Gathers
  - Organizes
  - Restores
  - Navigates

A

Impact on Client Factors (Body Functions and Structures)

- Sensory functions
  - Seeing functions
  Children with amblyopia may have to establish new habits and routines related to prescribed medical treatment involving patching.

Precautions

Early detection of amblyopia is important to prevent vision loss in the affected eye.

Evaluation

- Clinical observations
- Interviews with child and family
- Assessment tools

Suggested Assessment Tools

- Assessment of Motor and Process Skills (AMPS)
- Erhardt Developmental Vision Assessment, Revised (EDVA)
- School Assessment of Motor and Process Skills (School AMPS)
- School Function Assessment (SFA)

INTERVENTIONS

- Support for the child and family to develop habits and routines related to prescribed medical interventions
- Interventional support for the development of organizing space and objects
- Vision therapy, provided the occupational therapist has met the competencies for this advanced practice area

A

Case Example

Keisha is a first-grade student who is receiving medical treatment for amblyopia and often wears a patch during the school day according to the protocol prescribed by her doctor. Keisha's desk is disorganized, and now that her unaffected, stronger eye is patched, she finds it increasingly difficult to visually search for the items she needs. The occupational therapist works with Keisha to organize the materials in her desk so that they are easily accessible to her throughout the school day. ❖

WEB RESOURCES

American Association for Pediatric Ophthalmology and Strabismus
www.aapos.org

American Optometric Association
www.aoa.org/documents/CPG-4.pdf

FURTHER READING

Hartman E, Dobson V, Hainline L, et al: Preschool vision screenings: summary of a task force report, *Ophthalmology* 108:479, 2001.

8

❖

Anemia

Epidemiology

Anemia is a condition that is usually caused by an iron deficiency in the blood. It is diagnosed through blood tests and can usually be treated through an iron-rich nutrition program.

However, anemia can also be related to other conditions such as the following:

- Blood loss related to trauma
- Lead poisoning
- Chronic diseases
- Vitamin deficiencies
- Leukemia
- Sickle cell disease

It is estimated that approximately 20% of children in the United States will experience anemia some time during childhood.

Impact on Performance Skills

- Strength and effort
  - Moves
  - Transports
  - Lifts
  - Calibrates
  - Grips
- Energy

- Paces
- Attends

Impact on Client Factors (Body Functions and Structures)

Movement-related body structures and functions may be affected due to increased fatigue and decreased muscle strength. Children may also appear irritable and may complain of headaches.

Precautions

Children with anemia may need to develop new performance patterns to manage fatigue, take medication, and/or follow a nutritious diet.

Evaluation

- Clinical observations
- Interviews with child and family
- Assessment tools
- Manual muscle testing

Suggested Assessment Tools

- Assessment of Motor and Process Skills (AMPS)
- Bruininks-Oseretsky Test of Motor Performance (BOT-2)
- Miller Function and Participation Scales (M-FUN-S)
- Child Occupational Self Assessment (COSA)
- Perceived Efficacy and Goal Setting System (PEGS)
- Pediatric Activity Card Sort (PACS)

INTERVENTIONS

- Support for the child and family to develop habits and routines related to managing fatigue and prescribed medical interventions
- Energy conservation
- Strengthening and endurance

Case Example

Thomas is a 12-year-old boy who was recently admitted to the hospital to undergo chemotherapy treatment for leukemia. Thomas also has been diagnosed with anemia and reports increased fatigue. The nurses on the unit have been encouraging Thomas to get washed and dressed each morning, but Thomas frequently refuses. The occupational therapist works with Thomas to complete the COSA and finds out that although Thomas values such self-care activities, they are not important to him right now. Thomas would rather save his energy to talk and goof around with his friends when they come to visit. The occupational therapist supports Thomas in communicating this to the nursing staff and teaches him some energy conservation techniques. ❖

WEB RESOURCE

Nemours Foundation—Kids Health for Parents
www.kidshealth.org/parent/medical/heart/ida.html

FURTHER READING

Kohli-Kumar M: Screening for anemia in children: AAP recommendations—
    a critique, *Pediatrics* 108:1, 2001.

9

❖

Angelman Syndrome

Epidemiology

Angelman syndrome is a genetic disorder caused by the deletion of chromosome 15, mutation in the UBE3A gene, genetic imprinting defects, or other chromosomal defects.

It is estimated that approximately one in 10,000 to 20,000 individuals in the United States have Angelman syndrome.

Individuals with Angelman syndrome typically have developmental delays and intellectual disabilities. Motor delays and movement disorders are common, and children with Angelman syndrome typically have episodes of frequent and inappropriate laughter and/or hyperactivity.

Children with Angelman syndrome share unique facial characteristics such as the following:

- Wide mouths
- Widely spaced teeth
- Tendency to tongue thrust
- Prominent chin
- Squinting

Impact on Performance Skills

- Motor skills
  - Posture
  - Mobility
  - Coordination

A

- Strength and effort
- Energy
- Process skills
  - Energy
  - Knowledge
  - Temporal organization
  - Organizing space and objects
  - Adaptation
- Communication and interaction skills
  - Physicality
  - Information exchange
  - Relations

Impact on Client Factors (Body Functions and Structures)

- Global mental functions
- Specific mental functions
- Seeing functions (including strabismus)
- Functions of joints and bones
- Muscle functions
- Movement functions
- Voice and speech functions

Precautions

Children with Angelman syndrome may have seizure disorder.

Evaluation

- Clinical observations
- Interviews with child and family
- Assessment tools
- Manual muscle testing

Suggested Assessment Tools

- Alberta Infant Motor Scale (AIMS)
- Bayley Scale of Infant Development (BSID)

- Canadian Occupational Performance Measure (COPM)
- Children's Assessment of Participation and Enjoyment (CAPE)
- Denver Developmental Screening Test (DDST)
- Hawaii Early Learning Profile (HELP)
- Miller Function and Participation Scales (M-FUN-S)
- Peabody Developmental Motor Scales 2, Revised (PDMS-2)
- Pediatric Evaluation of Disability Inventory (PEDI)
- Pediatric Volitional Questionnaire (PVQ)
- School Function Assessment (SFA)
- Short Child Occupational Profile (SCOPE)
- Toddler and Infant Motor Evaluation (TIME)
- WeeFIM

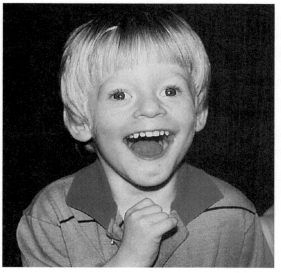

Angelman syndrome. (From Zitelli BJ, Davis HW: *Atlas of pediatric physical diagnosis,* ed 5, St Louis, 2007, Mosby.)

INTERVENTIONS

A

- Activities of daily living
- Instrumental activities of daily living
- Support for the development of independent leisure occupations
- Intervention to support the development of motor, process, and communication and interaction skills
- Accommodations and modifications for school and prevocational tasks

Case Example

Jim is a 10-year-old boy with Angelman syndrome. He is beginning to get dressed by himself in the morning but continues to struggle with fasteners, such as buttons and zippers. Jim's mother wants him to be able to dress independently and is afraid that if he gets frustrated he will give up. The occupational therapist recommends that Jim's mother set out clothes he can pull on that do not require increased fine motor dexterity. She also recommends slip-on athletic shoes so Jim does not have to tie them. ❖

WEB RESOURCES

Angelman Syndrome Foundation USA
www.angelman.org/angel

International Angelman Syndrome Organisation
www.asclepius.com/iaso

FURTHER READING

Walz N, Baranek G: Sensory processing patterns in persons with Angelman syndrome, *Am J Occup Ther* 60:472, 2006.

10

Anorexia

Epidemiology

Anorexia is a condition found in the *Diagnostic and Statistical Manual of Mental Disorders,* 4th Edition, Text Revision (DSM-IV-TR). It is characterized by an intense fear of becoming overweight and a poor and/or unrealistic body image. Individuals with anorexia are usually at least 25% underweight for their age and height.

Individuals with anorexia may restrict their caloric intact, engage in purging behavior (e.g., misusing laxatives or diuretics), or engage in both behaviors.

Anorexia is thought to be caused by a combination of psychologic, social, and physiologic factors.

Impact on Areas of Occupation
- Health management and maintenance
  - Presence of dominating habits and maladaptive routines

Impact on Performance Skills
- Strength and effort
  - Moves
  - Transports
  - Lifts
  - Calibrates
  - Grips

A

- Energy
  - Paces
  - Endures
  - Attends
- Knowledge
  - Heeds
- Temporal organization
  - Initiates
  - Continues
  - Sequences
  - Terminates
- Adaptation
  - Notices and responds
  - Accommodates
  - Adjusts
  - Benefits
- Relations
  - Conforms

Impact on Client Factors (Body Functions and Structures)

- Global mental functions
- Specific mental functions
  - Experience of self functions
- Neuromusculoskeletal and movement-related functions
- Cardiovascular system functions
- Respiratory system functions
- Digestive system functions
- Metabolic system and endocrine system functions

Precautions

Individuals with anorexia are at risk for developing numerous medical conditions, including organ failure.

Evaluation

- Clinical observations
- Interviews with child and family
- Assessment tools

Suggested Assessment Tools

- Adolescent Role Assessment (ARA)
- Behavior Assessment Rating Scale (BASC)
- Canadian Occupational Performance Measure (COPM)
- Child Behavior Checklist (CBCL)
- Interest Checklist
- Model of Human Occupation Screening Tool (MOHOST)
- NIH Activity Record
- Occupational Circumstances Assessment Interview and Rating Scale (OCAIRS)
- Occupational Performance History Interview (OPHI)

INTERVENTIONS

Cognitive behavioral therapy and metacognitive strategies leading to self-regulation (e.g., self-monitoring and self-evaluation)

Support to develop healthy habits and routines during activities of daily living (ADLs) and instrumental activities of daily living (IADLs)

Case Example

Elizabeth is a 16-year-old girl with anorexia who participates in an outpatient day treatment program for individuals with eating disorders. The occupational therapist helps Elizabeth to explore meal preparation of healthy food options that are a part of her nutritional program. ❖

WEB RESOURCE

Mayo Clinic
www.mayoclinic.com/health/anorexia/ds00606/dsection=2

FURTHER READING

Henderson S: Frames of reference utilized in the rehabilitation of individuals with eating disorders, *Can J Occup Ther* 66:43, 1999.

11

❖

Anxiety

Epidemiology

Anxiety is a sense of worry, apprehension, fear, or distress that is pervasive. Children with generalized anxiety disorder (GAD), a condition found in the *Diagnostic and Statistical Manual of Mental Disorders,* 4th Edition, Text Revision (DSM-IV-TR), experience anxiety and apprehension, as well as engaging in worrying most days within a 6-month period. GAD is thought to be caused by a combination of factors that include genetic predisposition, physiology, and psychologic concerns. In addition, GAD may be related to an associated medical condition.

Impact on Performance Skills

- Energy
  - Paces
  - Attends
- Temporal organization
  - Initiates
  - Continues
  - Sequences
  - Terminates
- Adaptation
  - Notices and responds
  - Accommodates
  - Adjusts

A

Impact on Client Factors (Body Functions and Structures)

- Digestive system functions (e.g., constipation or diarrhea, upset stomach)
- Global mental functions
  - Sleep
  - Temperament and personality functions
  - Energy and drive functions
- Specific mental functions
  - Attention functions
  - Memory functions
  - Thought functions

Precautions

GAD may be related to another medical or psychosocial condition.

Evaluation

- Clinical observations
- Interviews with child and family
- Assessment tools

Suggested Assessment Tools

- Assessment of Motor and Process Skills (AMPS)
- Adolescent Role Assessment (ARA)
- Behavior Assessment Rating Scale (BASC)
- Child Behavior Checklist (CBCL)
- Canadian Occupational Performance Measure (COPM)
- Coping Inventory
- Interest Checklist
- Model of Human Occupation Screening Tool (MOHOST)
- Occupational Circumstances Assessment Interview and Rating Scale (OCAIRS)
- Occupational Performance History Interview (OPHI)
- Pediatric Volitional Questionnaire (PVQ)

A

- School Assessment of Motor and Process Skills (School AMPS)
- Test of Everyday Attention for Children (TEA-Ch)
- Model of Human Occupation Screening Tool (MOHOST)
- The Occupational Circumstances Assessment Interview and Rating Scale (OCAIRS)

INTERVENTIONS

- Support for the development of habits and routines, including those related to sleep
- Support for coping with and reducing stressors
- Environmental accommodations and modifications
- Cognitive behavioral therapy and metacognitive strategies leading to self-regulation (e.g., self-monitoring and self-evaluation)
- Teaching of relaxation techniques

Case Example

Eric, a freshman in high school, has been diagnosed with GAD. Eric frequently worries about things that are out of his control and experiences a great deal of anxiety at school. As a result, he sometimes has difficulty paying attention in class and remembering to take down homework assignments. Eric's occupational therapist has been working with him to develop an organization system to assist him at school. In addition, she has recommended that Eric keep a journal. ❖

WEB RESOURCES

Anxiety Disorders Association of America
www.adaa.org

National Mental Health Association
www.nmha.org

FURTHER READING

Moffit T, Caspi A, Harrington H, et al: Generalized anxiety disorder and depression: childhood risk factors in a birth cohort followed to age 32, *Psychol Med* 37:441, 2007.

12

❖

Apnea

Epidemiology

Apnea is a pause in breathing during sleep that lasts for 20 seconds or longer. There are three types of apnea: obstructive, central, and mixed.

Obstructive apnea is caused by the obstruction of the airway, usually by tonsils or adenoids. Medical intervention for obstructive apnea sometimes includes the removal of the child's tonsils or adenoids. Signs and symptoms of obstructive apnea include the following:

- Snoring
- Mouth breathing
- Gasping for air
- Changes in color
- Frequent bedwetting
- Inability to remain asleep
- Irritability
- Tiredness
- Decreased attention during the day

Central apnea occurs when the center of the brain that controls breathing is not functioning properly. Central apnea is rare but more common in premature than full-term infants.

Mixed apnea is a combination of obstructive and central apnea.

Impact on Performance Skills

- Energy
- Knowledge
- Temporal organization
- Organization of spaces and objects
- Adaptation

Impact on Client Factors (Body Functions and Structures)

- Global mental functions
  - Sleep
  - Temperament and personality functions
  - Energy and drive functions
- Specific mental functions
  - Attention functions
  - Memory functions
  - Thought functions

Precautions

Parents and caregivers who suspect that their child has apnea should seek medical attention immediately. Children who are overweight are at greater risk for developing obstructive apnea.

Evaluation

- Clinical observations
- Interviews with child and family
- Assessment tools

Suggested Assessment Tools

- Assessment of Motor and Process Skills (AMPS)
- Bayley Scale of Infant Development (BSID)
- Denver Developmental Screening Test (DDST)
- FirstSTEp Developmental Screening Test
- Hawaii Early Learning Profile (HELP)
- McCarthy Scale of Children's Abilities
- Miller Assessment for Preschoolers (MAP)

- Peabody Developmental Motor Scales 2, Revised (PDMS-2)
- School Assessment of Motor and Process Skills (School AMPS)
- WeeFIM

INTERVENTIONS

- Recommendations of positions for sleep
- Caregiver education
- Classroom accommodations and modifications
- Exploration of interests related to physical activity

Case Example

Natalie is a 7-year-old girl who is overweight. Her mother reports that Natalie has been seen by a physician and has been diagnosed as having obstructive sleep apnea. Natalie frequently comes to school tired and struggles to remain awake after lunch. As a result, Natalie has difficulty attending to her afternoon lessons. The occupational therapist recommends that the teacher encourage Natalie to take frequent movement breaks throughout the afternoon so that she can maintain an arousal level appropriate for learning. ❖

WEB RESOURCES

Stanford—childhood apnea resource
www.stanford.edu/~dement/childapnea.html

Sleep Center at the Children's Hospital of Philadelphia
www.chop.edu/consumer/jsp/division/generic.jsp?id=71288

FURTHER READING

Schechter M: Technical report: diagnosis and management of childhood obstructive sleep apnea syndrome, *Pediatrics* 109:1, 2002.

13

❖

Arthrogryposis Multiplex Congenita

Epidemiology

Arthrogryposis affects approximately one in every 3000 infants and is characterized by multiple joint contractures, especially of the upper extremities and neck, at birth. Arthrogryposis is caused by decreased movement of the fetus in utero due to fetal abnormalities, such as issues related to connective tissue, or intrauterine trauma cause by maternal infection, illness, or drug use. The decreased fetal movement causes the development of extra connective tissue around joints, which then leads to contractures.

Individuals with arthrogryposis share common physical characteristics, such as the following:

• Pronounced joint rigidity
• Absent or diminished tendon reflexes
• Joint dislocation
• Soft-tissue webbing
• Scoliosis
• "Spindle-like" extremities that are absent of skin creases

Often the severity of joint rigidity will be increased distally.

Impact on Areas of Occupation

• Activities of daily living
• Instrumental activities of daily living

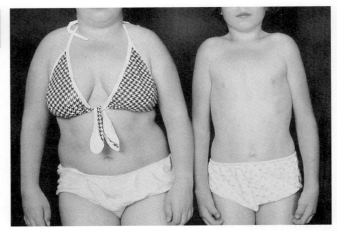

Arthrogryposis multiplex congenita. Note the stiff posture and tubular appearance of the limbs. Motion of all joints is limited as a result of failure in the development of or the degeneration of muscular structures. (From Zitelli BJ, Davis HW: *Atlas of pediatric physical diagnosis,* ed 5, St Louis, 2007, Mosby.)

- Education
- Work
- Play
- Leisure

Impact on Performance Skills

- Motor skills
  - Positions
  - Reaches
  - Bends
  - Coordinates
  - Manipulates
  - Flows
  - Moves
  - Transports
  - Lifts
  - Grips

A

- Energy
  - Endures
  - Paces

Impact on Client Factors (Body Functions and Structures)
- Functions of joints and bones
  - Mobility of joints
  - Mobility of bone functions
- Muscle functions
  - Muscle power functions
  - Muscle tone functions
  - Muscle endurance functions

Precautions
Individuals with arthrogryposis are prone to joint and bone fractures. Passive range-of-motion exercises should be performed only under the direction of the child's physician.

Evaluation
- Clinical observations
- Interviews with child and family
- Assessment tools

Suggested Assessment Tools
- Alberta Infant Motor Scale (AIMS)
- Assessment of Motor and Process Skills (AMPS)
- Bayley Scales of Infant Development (BSID)
- Canadian Occupational Performance Measure (COPM)
- Classroom Observation Guide
- Computer System Usability Questionnaire
- Denver Developmental Screening Test (DDST)
- Erhardt Developmental Prehension Assessment (EDPA)
- FirstSTEp Developmental Screening Test
- Hawaii Early Learning Profile (HELP)
- Home Observation and Measurement of the Environment (HOME)

A

- Knox Preschool Play Scale
- Motor Assessment Battery for Children (Movement ABC)
- Movement Assessment for Infants (MAI)
- Peabody Developmental Motor Scales 2, Revised (PDMS-2)
- Pediatric Evaluation of Disability Inventory (PEDI)
- School Assessment of Motor and Process Skills (School AMPS)
- School Function Assessment (SFA)
- School Setting Interview (SSI)
- Short Child Occupational Profile (SCOPE)
- Test of Environmental Supportiveness
- WeeFIM

INTERVENTIONS

- Interventions to support the development of posture, mobility, coordination, strength, and effort and to reduce contractures
- Support for occupational participation
- Environmental accommodations and modifications
- Task accommodations and modifications
- Caregiver and family coaching
- Assistive technology

Case Example

Phil is a 5-year-old with arthrogryposis who attends a half-day kindergarten program. The occupational therapist provides Phil with several pieces of assistive technology for him to use for self-feeding during snack time, such as a long-handled spoon and a cut-out cup. Phil and the occupational therapist are beginning to explore computer programs for him to use during journal time. ❖

WEB RESOURCES

National Support Group for Arthrogryposis Multiplex Congenita
www.avenuesforamc.com

National Organization for Rare Disorders
http://www.rarediseases.org

FURTHER READING

Bernstein R: Arthrogryposis and amyoplasia, *J Am Acad Orthop Surg* 10:417, 2002.

Hahn G: Arthrogryposis: pediatric review and habilitative aspects, *Clin Orthop Relat Res* 194:104, 1985.

A

14

❖

Asthma

Epidemiology

Asthma is a condition associated with the inflammation of the bronchial airways and causes increased mucus, mucosal swelling, and muscle contractions. Asthma has been linked to inflammation of the airway as a result of illness, allergies, infections, or exercise.

Common signs of asthma include coughing and wheezing, although not all children demonstrate these signs. Other signs and symptoms include shortness of breath and reports of tightness in the chest.

Impact on Performance Patterns

- Older children with asthma may need to develop routines related to medication management.
- Children may experience a decrease in role performance, or difficulty attaining new roles, owing to exacerbations.

Impact on Performance Skills

Asthma typically does not affect the development of performance skills except when the condition is severe. Motor-related performance skills may decline during an exacerbation. Exacerbations may be accompanied by decreased energy or endurance. In addition, if frequent school absences occur, children may require additional support to develop or maintain academic skills.

Impact on Client Factors (Body Functions and Structures)

- Respiratory system functions

Precautions

Exercise, infections, allergies, and irritants (e.g., perfume, tobacco smoke) may trigger an exacerbation. Children with frequent respiratory infections are at greater risk for asthma.

Evaluation

- Clinical observations
- Interviews with child and family
- Assessment tools

Suggested Assessment Tools

- Canadian Occupational Performance Measure (COPM)
- Child Occupational Self Assessment (COSA)
- Pediatric Activity Card Sort (PACS)
- Pediatric Interest Profile (PIP)
- Perceived Efficacy and Goal Setting System (PEGS)
- School Setting Interview (SSI)
- Short Child Occupational Profile (SCOPE)

INTERVENTIONS

- Interest exploration
- Role exploration
- Support for the development of habits and routines related to medication management
- Education for child about signs and symptoms of an exacerbation
- Environmental modifications (e.g., reduction of irritants)
- School accommodations
- Leisure-related accommodations and modifications

A

*Case Example*_____

Tom, a child with asthma, will be entering high school next year and would like to assume the role of a member on a sports team. Owing to frequent exacerbations during elementary school, Tom did not have the opportunity to play on a team. The occupational therapist works with Tom to explore his interests related to sports and helps him select a team to try out for. ❖

WEB RESOURCES

American Lung Association
www.lungusa.org/site/pp.asp?c=dvluk9o0e&b=22782

Asthma and Allergy Association of America
www.aafa.org/display.cfm?id=8&sub=16&cont=44

FURTHER READING

Chiang L, Huang J, Fu L: Physical activity and physical self-concept: comparison between children with and without asthma, *J Adv Nurs* 54:653, 2006.

15

❖

Attention Deficit/ Hyperactivity Disorder

Epidemiology

Attention deficit/hyperactivity disorder (ADHD) is classified in the *Diagnostic and Statistical Manual of Mental Disorders,* 4th Edition, Text Revision (DSM-IV-TR); such disorders are estimated to affect approximately 5% to 10% of children. There are three subtypes of ADHD. They include the following:

- Predominantly hyperactive-impulsive type, which does not include significant inattention
- Predominantly inattentive type, which does not include significant hyperactive or impulsive behavior
- Combined type, which means that the child demonstrates hyperactive-impulsive and inattentive behaviors

ADHD may be caused by medical disorders or conditions that affect brain functioning of sensory functions, anxiety or depression, sudden changes in the child's life, or learning disabilities. For a child to be diagnosed with ADHD, he or she must meet the criteria established in the DSM-IV-TR. Symptoms of ADHD must:

- Appear before the age of 7 years
- Continue at least 6 months

- Greatly affect the child's ability to participate at home, at school, and in the community

Impact on Performance Skills

- Knowledge
  - Chooses
  - Uses
  - Handles
  - Heeds
  - Inquires
- Temporal organization
  - Initiates
  - Continues
  - Sequences
  - Terminates
- Organization of space and objects
  - Searches and locates
  - Gathers
  - Organizes
  - Restores
  - Navigates
- Adaptation
  - Notices and responds
  - Accommodates
  - Adjusts
- Physicality
  - Contacts
  - Maneuvers
- Information exchange
  - Expresses
  - Modulates
- Relations
  - Collaborates
  - Conforms
  - Focuses
  - Relates
  - Respects

Impact on Client Factors (Body Functions and Structures)

A

- Global mental functions
  - Sleep
  - Temperament and personality functions
  - Energy and drive functions
- Specific mental functions
  - Attention functions
  - Memory functions
  - Thought functions
- Sensory functions

Precautions

Children with ADHD may sometimes engage in dangerous and risky behavior owing to difficulty with impulse control.

Evaluation

- Clinical observations
- Interviews with child and family
- Assessment tools

Suggested Assessment Tools

- Assessment of Motor and Process Skills (AMPS)
- Canadian Occupational Performance Measure (COPM)
- Child and Adolescent Social Perception Measure
- Child Occupational Self Assessment (COSA)
- Children's Paced Auditory Serial Addition Test (CHIPASAT)
- Coping Inventory
- Dynamic Occupational Therapy Cognitive Assessment for Children (DOTCA-Ch)
- Knox Cube Test
- Lowenstein Occupational Therapy Cognitive Assessment (LOTCA)
- McCarthy Scale of Children's Abilities
- Miller Assessment for Preschoolers (MAP)

A

- Miller Function and Participation Scales (M-FUN-S)
- Perceived Efficacy and Goal Setting System (PEGS)
- School Assessment of Motor and Process Skills (School AMPS)
- School Function Assessment (SFA)
- School Setting Interview (SSI)
- Short Child Occupational Profile (SCOPE)
- Social Skills Rating System
- Test of Everyday Attention for Children (TEA-Ch)

INTERVENTIONS

- Environmental accommodations and modifications
- Task accommodations and modifications
- Interventions to support the development of self-regulatory skills
- Interventions to increase the following:
  - Safety awareness
  - Knowledge
  - Temporal organization
  - Organization of space and objects
  - Adaptation
  - Physicality
  - Information exchange
- Social skills training
- Caregiver and family coaching
- Intervention to support routines related to organization

Case Example

Will is a fourth-grade student with a diagnosis of ADHD, predominantly hyperactive-impulsive type. Will has difficulty remaining still and paying attention at school. The occupational therapist provides education to Will's general education teacher about his condition, and with Will's input they develop a schedule for movement breaks throughout the day. In addition, Will and the occupational therapist work together to develop an organizational system for Will's school materials. ❖

WEB RESOURCES

Attention Deficit Disorder Association
www.add.org

Children and Adults with Attention Deficit Disorder
www.chadd.org

FURTHER READING

White B, Mulligan SE: Behavioral and physiologic response measures of occupational task performance: a preliminary comparison between typical children and children with attention disorder, *Am J Occup Ther* 59:426, 2005.

16

❖

Autism Spectrum Disorders

Epidemiology

Autism spectrum disorders (ASDs) are a group of five developmental disabilities that occur in all racial and ethnic groups. ASDs are four times more likely to occur in boys than in girls, except for Rett's syndrome. It is estimated that approximately one in 150 children in the United States has an ASD. Although a great deal of research is being done to find the cause of ASD, no definitive cause has been established. The five types of ASDs are classified in the *Diagnostic and Statistical Manual of Mental Disorders,* 4th Edition, Text Revision (DSM-IV-TR). Children with ASDs have variable presentations.

Autistic Disorder

Autistic disorder is characterized by an onset before age three. Children with autistic disorder typically have the following indicators:
- Qualitative impairment in social interaction, which may include the following:
  - Eye contact
  - Facial expression
  - Body postures
  - Gestures
  - Failure to develop peer relationships
  - Lack of spontaneous initiation
  - Lack of social or emotional reciprocity

- Qualitative impairment in communication, which may include the following:
  - Delay in development or lack of spoken language
  - Marked impairment in ability to sustain conversations
  - Stereotyped or repetitive use of language
  - Lack of social imitative play
- Restricted repetitive and stereotyped patterns of behavior, interests, and activities, such as the following:
  - Inflexible adherence to routines or rituals
  - Stereotyped or repetitive motor movements
  - Preoccupation with parts of objects

Pervasive Developmental Disorder—Not Otherwise Specified

Pervasive developmental disorder—not otherwise specified (PDD-NOS) is characterized by a severe and pervasive impairment in social reciprocity and interaction as evidenced by an impairment in verbal and/or nonverbal communication skills. Children with PDD-NOS may also engage in stereotyped behaviors or patterns of interest. They do not meet the criteria for any other ASD.

Asperger's Syndrome

Asperger's syndrome is different from autistic disorder or "high-functioning autism." Individuals with Asperger's syndrome typically have the following indicators:

- Developmentally appropriate language abilities
- Developmentally appropriate intellectual abilities
- Qualitative impairment in social interaction characterized by the following:
  - Marked impairment in the use of multiple nonverbal behaviors
  - Failure to develop peer relationships appropriate to developmental level
  - Lack of spontaneous social interactions
  - Lack of social or emotional reciprocity

- Restricted repetitive and stereotyped patterns of behavior, interests, and activities characterized by the following:
  - A preoccupation with one or more stereotyped and restricted patterns of interest that is abnormal in intensity of focus
  - Inflexible adherence to routines or rituals
  - Stereotyped and repetitive motor mannerisms
  - Persistent preoccupation with parts of objects

Rett's Syndrome

Rett's syndrome is characterized by typical development through the fifth month of life. Between the ages of five months and 48 months the child experiences a deceleration of head growth and a loss of hand skills. Individuals with Rett's syndrome engage in characteristic repetitive movement that looks like hand-washing or hand-wringing and may have decreased expressive and receptive language development and poorly coordinated gait and trunk movements. Rett's syndrome is more common in girls.

Childhood Disintegrative Disorder

Childhood disintegrative disorder is characterized by typical development during the first 2 years of life and a significant loss of acquired skills, such as expressive or receptive language, social skills, adaptive behavior, bowel and bladder management, play skills, or motor skills. It is also characterized by the following:

- Qualitative impairment in social interaction, which may include the following:
  - Eye contact
  - Facial expression
  - Body postures
  - Gestures
  - Failure to develop peer relationships
  - Lack of spontaneous initiation
  - Lack of social or emotional reciprocity

A

- Qualitative impairment in communication, which may include the following:
  - A delay in development of or lack of spoken language
  - Marked impairment of ability to sustain conversations
  - Stereotyped or repetitive use of language
  - Lack of social imitative play
- Restricted repetitive and stereotyped patterns of behavior, interests, and activities, such as the following:
  - Inflexible adherence to routines or rituals
  - Stereotyped or repetitive motor movements
  - Preoccupation with parts of objects

Impact on Areas of Occupation
- Activities of daily living
- Instrumental activities of daily living
- Education
- Play
- Leisure
- Social interaction

Impact on Performance Patterns
- Restricted patterns of interest
- Limited roles
- Dominating habits

Impact on Performance Skills
- Mobility
- Coordination
- Strength and effort
- Energy
- Knowledge
- Temporal organization
- Organization of space and objects
- Adaptation
- Physicality
- Information exchange
- Relations

Impact on Client Factors (Body Functions and Structures)

A

- Global mental functions
- Specific mental functions
- Sensory functions
- Movement functions
- Voice and speech functions

Precautions

No precautions have been noted.

Evaluation

- Clinical observations
- Interviews with child and family
- Assessment tools

Suggested Assessment Tools

- Assessment of Motor and Process Skills (AMPS)
- Canadian Occupational Performance Measure (COPM)
- Child and Adolescent Social Perception Measure
- Child Occupational Self Assessment (COSA)
- Children's Assessment of Participation and Enjoyment (CAPE)
- Coping Inventory
- Dynamic Occupational Therapy Cognitive Assessment for Children (DOTCA-Ch)
- Infant/Toddler Sensory Profile
- Knox Cube Test
- Lowenstein Occupational Therapy Cognitive Assessment (LOTCA)
- McCarthy Scale of Children's Abilities
- Miller Assessment for Preschoolers (MAP)
- Miller Function and Participation Scales (M-FUN-S)
- Pediatric Volitional Questionnaire (PVQ)
- Perceived Efficacy and Goal Setting System (PEGS)
- Play History

A

- Playform
- Preferences for Activities of Children (PAC)
- Preschool and Kindergarten Behavior Scales (PKBS)
- School Assessment of Motor and Process Skills (School AMPS)
- School Function Assessment (SFA)
- School Sensory Profile
- School Setting Interview (SSI)
- Sensory Processing Measure (SPM)
- Sensory Profile
- Short Child Occupational Profile (SCOPE)
- Social Skills Rating System
- Test of Environmental Supportiveness
- Test of Everyday Attention for Children (TEA-Ch)
- Test of Playfulness
- Vineland Adaptive Behavior Scales Revised (VABS)

INTERVENTIONS

- Activities of daily living
- Instrumental activities of daily living
- Educational accommodations and modifications
- Community-oriented accommodations and modifications
- Play skills
- Self-regulation
- Development of useful habits and routines
- Role exploration
- Interventions to develop functional communication and interaction skills
- Staff and caregiver education and training
- Sensory processing
- Support for volitional development
- Behavior management
- Motor skill development
- Process skill development
- Prevocational skills

Case Example

Ben is a 4-year-old with PDD child who attends an early child-hood education program. The occupational therapist works with the classroom teacher to ensure that Ben has access to visual supports, such as a timer and picture schedule, for transitions. ❖

A

WEB RESOURCES

Centers for Disease Control and Prevention
www.cdc.gov/ncbddd/autism/ActEarly/autism.html

Autism Speaks
www.autismspeaks.org

FURTHER READING

Watling R, Tomcheck S, LaVesser P: The scope of occupational therapy services for individuals with autism spectrum disorders across the lifespan, *Am J Occup Ther* 59:680, 2005.

17

❖

Bipolar Disorder

Epidemiology

Bipolar disorder is a condition classified in the *Diagnostic and Statistical Manual of Mental Disorders,* 4th Edition, Text Revision (DSM-IV-TR) and is characterized by extreme changes in mood, energy, thinking, and behavior. Children who have been diagnosed with bipolar disorder may experience symptoms in early childhood, or symptoms may emerge in adolescence or adulthood.

Symptoms of bipolar disorder include marked changes in mood or energy, extreme sadness, rapid changes in mood, destructive rages, separation anxiety, hyperactivity and distractibility, disrupted sleep patterns, impaired judgment and safety awareness, and illogical beliefs related to one's own abilities.

Impact on Performance Skills

- Knowledge
  - Chooses
  - Uses
  - Handles
  - Heeds
  - Inquires
- Temporal organization
  - Initiates
  - Continues

B

- Sequences
- Terminates
- Organization of space and objects
  - Searches and locates
  - Gathers
  - Organizes
  - Restores
  - Navigates
- Adaptation
  - Notices and responds
  - Accommodates
  - Adjusts
- Physicality
  - Contacts
  - Maneuvers
- Information exchange
  - Expresses
  - Modulates
- Relations
  - Collaborates
  - Conforms
  - Focuses
  - Relates
  - Respects

Impact on Client Factors (Body Functions and Structures)

- Global mental functions
  - Sleep
  - Temperament and personality functions
  - Energy and drive functions
- Specific mental functions
  - Attention functions
  - Memory functions
  - Thought functions

Precautions

Children who have been diagnosed with bipolar disorder may be taking medication. Occupational therapists should carefully monitor changes in mood and occupational performance and share this information with the child's family and physician as appropriate. Any child who discusses or otherwise indicates suicidal thoughts or behaviors should be taken seriously. Children with bipolar disorder are also at risk for engaging in dangerous or risky behavior.

Evaluation

- Clinical observations
- Interviews with child and family
- Assessment tools

Suggested Assessment Tools

- Assessment of Motor and Process Skills (AMPS)
- Canadian Occupational Performance Measure (COPM)
- Child and Adolescent Social Perception Measure
- Child Occupational Self Assessment (COSA)
- Dynamic Occupational Therapy Cognitive Assessment for Children (DOTCA-Ch)
- Lowenstein Occupational Therapy Cognitive Assessment (LOTCA)
- Miller Function and Participation Scales (M-FUN-S)
- Pediatric Volitional Questionnaire (PVQ)
- Perceived Efficacy and Goal Setting System (PEGS)
- School Assessment of Motor and Process Skills (School AMPS)
- School Function Assessment (SFA)
- School Setting Interview (SSI)
- Short Child Occupational Profile (SCOPE)
- Social Skills Rating System
- Test of Everyday Attention for Children (TEA-Ch)

INTERVENTIONS

- Support for the development of habits and routines
- Support for coping with and reducing stressors
- Environmental accommodations and modification
- Cognitive behavioral therapy and metacognitive strategies leading to self-regulation (e.g., self-monitoring and self-evaluation)
- Teaching of relaxation techniques
- Addressing of occupational performance in activites of daily living, IADLS, education, play, leisure, and social and community participation
- Family and caregiver training and education
- Role exploration
- Prevocational skills training

Case Example

Alicia is a 17-year-old girl who has been diagnosed with bipolar disorder. Alicia is working with the occupational therapist to develop skills related to interviewing and exploring policies related to disclosing disability in the workplace. ❖

WEB RESOURCES

Child and Adolescent Bipolar Foundation
www.bpkids.org

National Alliance on Mental Illness
www.nami.org

FURTHER READING

Chang K, Howe M, Gallelli K, Miklowitz D: Prevention of pediatric bipolar disorder: integration of neurobiological and psychosocial process, *Ann N Y Acad Sci* 1094:235, 2006.

18

❖

Brachial Plexus Injury

Epidemiology

Brachial plexus injuries often occur during birth as a result of excessive traction and shoulder dystocia. Brachial plexus injuries are caused by damage to nerves that come from the spinal cord and control muscle movement and sensation in the shoulder, arm, and hand. Infants with minor injuries often do not require medical intervention. However, those who incur more traumatic injuries may require intensive intervention and possibly surgery to regain function in the affected upper extremity.

Other terms commonly used to describe brachial plexus injuries include *Erb's palsy* (upper trunk injury), *Klumpke's palsy* (lower trunk injury), *brachial plexus palsy, Erb-Duchenne palsy, Horner's syndrome* (when facial nerves are also affected), and *"burners"* or *"stingers"* (usually associated with sports-related brachial plexus injuries).

Three common types of brachial plexus injuries in the order of least to most severe are as follows:

- Stretch of the nerve
- Rupture of the nerve
- Avulsion of the nerve

Impact on Performance Skills

- Mobility
- Coordination
- Strength and effort

B

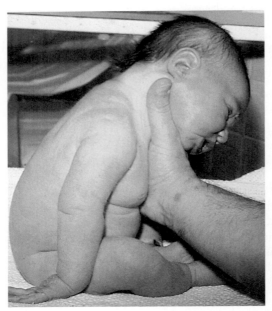

Brachial plexus injury. A traction injury to C5, C6, and C7 spinal cord segments produces this Erb palsy. (From Zitelli BJ, Davis HW: *Atlas of pediatric physical diagnosis,* ed 5, St Louis, 2007, Mosby.)

Impact on Client Factors (Body Functions and Structures)

- Sensation functions
- Movement functions
- Muscle functions

Precautions

Extra care should be taken during range-of-motion exercises and when moving the infant or child to prevent further injury.

Evaluation

- Clinical observations, including active range of motion (AROM), active assistive range of motion
- (AAROM), and passive range of motion (PROM)
- Interviews with child and family
- Assessment tools

Suggested Assessment Tools

- Alberta Infant Motor Scale (AIMS)
- Bayley Scale of Infant Development (BSID)
- Canadian Occupational Performance Measure (COPM)
- Children's Assessment of Participation and Enjoyment (CAPE)
- Denver Developmental Screening Test (DDST)
- Hawaii Early Learning Profile (HELP)
- Miller Function and Participation Scales (M-FUN-S)
- Peabody Developmental Motor Scales 2, Revised (PDMS-2)
- Pediatric Evaluation of Disability Inventory (PEDI)
- School Function Assessment (SFA)
- School Setting Interview (SSI)
- Short Child Occupational Profile (SCOPE)
- Toddler and Infant Motor Evaluation (TIME)
- WeeFIM

INTERVENTIONS

- Interventions to support the development of coordination, strength, and effort
- Support for participation in self-care and play
- Environmental accommodations and modifications
- Task accommodations and modifications
- Caregiver and family coaching

Case Example

The occupational therapist is working with Mrs. Jones and her 1-month-old infant, who acquired a brachial plexus injury during birth. The occupational therapist coaches the mother on how to pick up and hold the infant after surgery. ❖

WEB RESOURCES

Mayo Clinic
www.mayoclinic.org

Brachial Plexus Foundation
www.brachialplexuspalsyfoundation.org

FURTHER READING

DiTaranto P, Campagna L, Price A, Grossman JA: Outcome following non-operative treatment of brachial plexus birth injuries, *J Child Neurol* 19:87, 2004.

19

❖

Bronchopulmonary Dysplasia

Epidemiology

Bronchopulmonary dysplasia (BPD) is a common respiratory condition found in infants who were born prematurely and is caused by progressive lung inflammation. It is estimated that 5000 to 10,000 cases of BPD are reported annually in the United States. Children who are born weighing less than 1000 g (2.2 lb) are at greater risk for developing BPD.

Medical treatment for BPD involves supporting the breathing and oxygen needs of the infants. Infants with BPD may be treated with bronchodilators or ventilators. They may also receive their nutrition through intravenous feedings.

Impact on Occupational Performance

All co-occupations related to the infant and his or her caregivers are affected by BPD, including bathing, dressing, changing, feeding, and social interactions.

Impact on Performance Patterns

Infants who are receiving services in the neonatal intensive care unit (NICU) may experience disturbances in their natural rhythms and routines.

Impact on Client Factors (Body Functions and Structures)

- Respiratory system functions
- Cardiovascular system functions

Precautions

Infants with BPD are at greater risk for contracting respiratory infections such as pneumonia. Complications related to BPD can be fatal.

Evaluation

- Clinical observations
- Interviews with family and nursing staff
- Caregiver questionnaires and checklists

INTERVENTIONS

- Support for the volitional development of new parents and caregivers in the NICU
- Support for the development of caregiver-infant co-occupations
- Infant positioning
- Environmental modifications
- Caregiver education and coaching
- Staff training

Case Example

Rafael is a premature infant with an adjusted age of 1 week. The occupational therapist educates Rafael's parents about BPD. Together they identify ways that Rafael's parents can be more involved with his care. ❖

WEB RESOURCE

American Lung Association
www.lungusa.org

FURTHER READING

Vegara E, Anzalone M, Bigsby R, et al: Specialized knowledge and skills for occupational therapy practice in the neonatal intensive care unit, *Am J Occup Ther* 60:659, 2006.

B

20

❖

Bulimia

Epidemiology

Bulimia is an eating disorder found in the *Diagnostic and Statistical Manual of Mental Disorders,* 4th Edition, Text Revision (DSM-IV-TR). Bulimia is characterized by excessive secretive eating followed by inappropriate methods of weight control. Individuals with bulimia may purge by vomiting, misusing laxatives and diuretics, and/or engaging in excessive exercise. In addition, individuals with bulimia have distorted body images. It is estimated that approximately 3% of all women in the United States have experienced bulimia.

Impact on Areas of Occupation

Because of the presence of dominating habits and maladaptive routines, many areas of occupational participation may be affected, including the following:
- Health management and maintenance
- Activities of daily living
- Instrumental activities of daily living
- Social participation

Impact on Performance Skills

Specific performance skills may not be affected; however, because the cycle of binging and purging is typically done in secret, individuals with bulimia may at times struggle with appropriate communication and interaction skills.

Impact on Client Factors (Body Functions and Structures)

Individuals with bulimia put themselves at greater risk for digestive and metabolic system dysfunctions. Individuals who purge by vomiting are at risk for esophageal ulcers, ruptures, or strictures. In addition, they may have poor dentition from abnormal exposure to gastric acids. The misuse of diuretics can cause edema, and regular use of laxatives can negatively affect the function of the colon.

Other functions and structures affected include the following:
- Cardiovascular system functions
- Global mental functions
- Specific mental functions
  - Experience of self functions

Precautions

Individuals with bulimia are at risk for developing numerous associated medical conditions.

Evaluation
- Clinical observations
- Interviews with child and family
- Assessment tools

Suggested Assessment Tools
- Adolescent Role Assessment (ARA)
- Assessment of Motor and Process Skills (AMPS)
- Canadian Occupational Performance Measure (COPM)
- Coping Inventory
- Experience of Leisure Scale (TELS)
- Interest Checklist
- Leisure Competence Measure
- Model of Human Occupation Screening Tool (MOHOST)
- NIH Activity Record

- Occupational Circumstances Assessment Interview and Rating Scale (OCAIRS)
- Occupational Performance History Interview (OPHI)
- Pediatric Interest Profile (PIP)
- Volitional Questionnaire

INTERVENTIONS

- Cognitive behavioral therapy and metacognitive strategies leading to self-regulation (e.g., self-monitoring and self-evaluation)
- Support to develop healthy habits and routines during areas of occupational participation

Case Example

Jody is a 15-year-old girl with bulimia who was recently admitted to an inpatient unit. Jody attends a weekly goal-setting group as part of occupational therapy. During the group she chooses goals to work on during the next week, as well as how she will monitor her progress and evaluate her outcome at the end of the week. Sometimes Jody's goals relate to nutrition or fitness; at other times they focus on positive body image and asserting herself. ❖

WEB RESOURCES

Academy for Eating Disorders
www.aedweb.org

National Eating Disorders Association
www.nationaleatingdisorders.org/p.asp?WebPage_ID=337

FURTHER READING

Schmidt U, Lee S, Beecham J, et al: A randomized controlled trial of family therapy and cognitive behavior therapy guided self-care for adolescents with bulimia nervosa and related disorders, *Am J Psychiatr* 164:591, 2007.

21

❖

Cerebral Palsy

Epidemiology

Cerebral palsy (CP) is a broad term that encompasses several neurologic disorders that occur at birth or in early infancy. CP affects movement, muscle tone, and coordination. It is caused by an insult or injury to the fetus's or infant's brain and can be caused by any of the following: illness, injury or inflammation of the brain, abnormal brain development, severe jaundice, cerebrovascular incident, or anoxia.

Approximately two or three children out of 1000 will be affected by CP. Most will be born with noticeable signs, and all should be diagnosed by age 3.

CP can affect part or all of the body and is described with the following terms:

- *Diplegia:* primarily affecting the lower extremities
- *Hemiplegia:* primarily affecting the upper extremity and lower extremity of one side of the body
- *Quadriplegia:* affecting bilateral upper and bilateral lower extremities, sometimes including the trunk

CP is also classified by the quality of motor movement and is described with the following terms:

- *Spastic:* high tone characterized by tight, rigid muscles
- *Athetoid:* fluctuating muscle tone and writhing movements
- *Ataxic:* characterized by lack of coordination with intentional movements

C

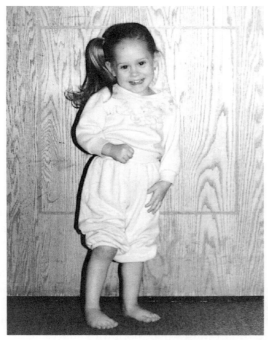

Cerebral palsy. (From Zitelli BJ, Davis HW: *Atlas of pediatric physical diagnosis,* ed 5, St Louis, 2007, Mosby.)

- *Hypotonic:* low tone, loose muscles, and lax joints
- *Mixed:* a combination of two or more of the above

Finally, CP is classified functionally. The Manual Ability Classification System (MACS) (Table 21-1) and Gross Motor Function Classification System (GMFCS) (Table 21-2) are both used to describe the impact of CP on how children functionally use their bodies to participate in daily occupations.

Impact on Performance Skills

- Motor skills
  - Posture
  - Mobility

TABLE 21-1
Manual Ability Classification System

Level	Description
I	Handles objects easily and successfully
II	Handles most objects but with somewhat reduced quality and/or speed of achievement
III	Handles objects with difficulty; needs help to prepare and/or modify activities
IV	Handles a limited selection of easily managed objects in adapted situations
V	Does not handle objects and has severely limited ability to perform even simple actions

Adapted from Eliasson AC, Krumlinde-Sundholm L, Rösblad B, et al: The Manual Ability Classification System (MACS) for children with cerebral palsy: scale development and evidence of validity and reliability, *Dev Med Child Neurol* 48:549, 2006.

- Coordination
- Strength and effort
- Energy
- Communication and interaction skills
  - Physicality
    - Gestures
    - Postures
  - Information exchange
    - Is articulate
    - Speaks
    - Sustains

Impact on Client Factors (Body Functions and Structures)

- Neuromusculoskeletal and movement-related functions
  - Muscle functions
  - Movement functions
- Voice and speech functions

TABLE 21-2

Gross Motor Function Classification System for Cerebral Palsy

Level	Description
Before Second Birthday	
I	Infants move in and out of sitting and floor sit with both hands free to manipulate objects. Infants crawl on hands and knees, pull to stand, and take steps while holding onto furniture. Infants walk between 18 months and 2 years of age without the need for any assistive mobility device.
II	Infants maintain floor sitting but may need to use their hands for support to maintain balance. Infants creep on their stomachs or crawl on hands and knees. Infants may pull to stand and take steps while holding onto furniture.
III	Infants maintain floor sitting when the low back is supported. Infants roll and creep forward on their stomachs.
IV	Infants have head control, but trunk support is required for floor sitting. Infants can roll to supine and may roll to prone positions.
V	Physical impairments limit voluntary control of movement. Infants are unable to maintain antigravity head and trunk postures in prone and sitting positions. Infants require adult assistance to roll.
Between Second and Fourth Birthdays	
I	Children floor sit with both hands free to manipulate objects. Movements in and out of floor sitting and standing are performed without adult assistance. Children walk as the preferred method of mobility without the need for any assistive mobility device.

C

II   Children floor sit but may have difficulty with balance when both hands are free to manipulate objects. Movements in and out of sitting are performed without adult assistance. Children pull to stand on a stable surface. Children crawl on hands and knees with a reciprocal pattern, cruise while holding onto furniture, and walk using an assistive mobility device as preferred methods of mobility.

III   Children maintain floor sitting often by "W-sitting" (sitting between flexed and internally rotated hips and knees) and may require adult assistance to assume sitting position. Children creep on their stomachs or crawl on hands and knees (often without reciprocal leg movements) as their primary methods of self-mobility. Children may pull on a stable surface to stand and may cruise short distances. Children may walk short distances indoors using an assistive mobility device and adult assistance for steering and turning.

IV   Children floor sit when placed but are unable to maintain alignment and balance without use of their hands for support. Children frequently require adaptive equipment for sitting and standing. Self-mobility for short distances (within a room) is achieved through rolling, creeping on stomach, or crawling on hands and knees without reciprocal leg movement.

V   Physical impairments restrict voluntary control of movement and the ability to maintain antigravity head and trunk postures. All areas of motor function are limited. Functional limitations in sitting and standing are not fully compensated for through the use of adaptive equipment and assistive technology. At level V, children have no means of independent mobility and are transported. Some children achieve self-mobility using a power wheelchair with extensive adaptations.

TABLE 21-2

Gross Motor Function Classification System for Cerebral Palsy—cont'd

Level	Description
Between Fourth and Sixth Birthdays	
I	Children get into and out of, and sit in, a chair without the need for hand support. Children move from the floor and from chair sitting to standing without the need for objects for support. Children walk indoors and outdoors and climb stairs. Children demonstrate an emerging ability to run and jump.
II	Children sit in a chair with both hands free to manipulate objects. Children move from the floor to standing and from chair sitting to standing but often require a stable surface to push or pull up on with their arms. Children walk without the need for any assistive mobility device indoors and for short distances on level surfaces outdoors. Children climb stairs holding onto a railing but are unable to run or jump.
III	Children sit on a regular chair but may require pelvic or trunk support to maximize hand function. Children move into and out of chair sitting using a stable surface to push on or pull up with their arms. Children walk with an assistive mobility device on level surfaces and climb stairs with assistance from an adult. Children frequently are transported when traveling for long distances or outdoors on uneven terrain.

IV   Children sit on a chair but need adaptive seating for trunk control and to maximize hand function. Children move into and out of chair sitting with assistance from an adult or a stable surface to push or pull up on with their arms. Children may at best walk short distances with a walker and adult supervision but have difficulty turning and maintaining balance on uneven surfaces. Children are transported in the community. Children may achieve self-mobility using a power wheelchair.

V   Physical impairments restrict voluntary control of movement and the ability to maintain antigravity head and trunk postures. All areas of motor function are limited. Functional limitations in sitting and standing are not fully compensated for through the use of adaptive equipment and assistive technology. At level V, children have no means of independent mobility and are transported. Some children achieve self-mobility using a power wheelchair with extensive adaptations.

Between Sixth and Twelfth Birthdays

I   Children walk indoors and outdoors and climb stairs without limitations. Children perform gross motor skills including running and jumping, but speed, balance, and coordination are reduced.

II   Children walk indoors and outdoors and climb stairs holding onto a railing but experience limitations walking on uneven surfaces and inclines and walking in crowds or confined spaces. Children have at best only minimal ability to perform gross motor skills such as running and jumping.

TABLE 21-2

Gross Motor Function Classification System for Cerebral Palsy—cont'd

Level	Description
III	Children walk indoors or outdoors on a level surface with an assistive mobility device. Children may climb stairs holding onto a railing. Depending on upper limb function, children propel a wheelchair manually or are transported when traveling for long distances or outdoors on uneven terrain.
IV	Children may maintain levels of function achieved before age 6 or may rely more on wheeled mobility at home, in school, and in the community. Children may achieve self-mobility using a power wheelchair.
V	Physical impairments restrict voluntary control of movement and the ability to maintain antigravity head and trunk postures. All areas of motor function are limited. Functional limitations in sitting and standing are not fully compensated for through the use of adaptive equipment and assistive technology. At level V, children have no means of independent mobility and are transported. Some children achieve self-mobility using a power wheelchair with extensive adaptations.

From Palisano R, Rosenbaum P, Walter S, et al: Development and reliability of a system to classify gross motor function in children with cerebral palsy, *Dev Med Child Neurol* 39:214, 1997.

Precautions
Some children with CP have other medical conditions that affect them on daily basis, such as seizure disorder.

Evaluation
- Clinical observations
- Interviews with child and family
- Assessment tools

Suggested Assessment Tools
- Alberta Infant Motor Scale (AIMS)
- Assessment of Motor and Process Skills (AMPS)
- Bayley Scale of Infant Development (BSID)
- Canadian Occupational Performance Measure (COPM)
- Classroom Observation Guide
- Child Occupational Self Assessment (COSA)
- Children's Assessment of Participation and Enjoyment (CAPE)
- Coping Inventory
- Denver Developmental Screening Test (DDST)
- Erhardt Developmental Prehension Assessment (EDPA)
- Evaluation Tool of Children's Handwriting (ETCH)
- Gross Motor Function Measure (GMFM)
- Hawaii Early Learning Profile (HELP)
- Miller Assessment for Preschoolers (MAP)
- Miller Function and Participation Scales (M-FUN-S)
- Peabody Developmental Motor Scales 2, Revised (PDMS-2)
- Pediatric Evaluation of Disability Inventory (PEDI)
- Pediatric Interest Profile (PIP)
- Pediatric Volitional Questionnaire (PVQ)
- School Assessment of Motor and Process Skills (School AMPS)
- School Function Assessment (SFA)
- School Setting Interview (SSI)
- Short Child Occupational Profile (SCOPE)
- Toddler and Infant Motor Evaluation (TIME)
- WeeFIM

INTERVENTIONS

- Activities of daily living
- Instrumental activities of daily living
- Education
- Leisure
- Accommodations and modifications
- Support for the development of muscle strength and motor function
- Support for the development of motor and communication and interaction skills
- Tone management
- Assistive technology and adaptive equipment
- Family coaching and training
- Support for the development of self-determination skills
- Support for the development of prevocational skills

Case Example

Lucy is a 12-year-old girl with spastic quadriplegia. Lucy drives a power wheelchair and uses a communication device. The occupational therapist is working with her on coaching her personal care assistant. ❖

WEB RESOURCES

United Cerebral Palsy
www.ucp.org

Gross Motor Function Classification System (GMFCS)
www.canchild.ca/Portals/0/outcomes/pdf/GMFCS.pdf

Manual Ability Classification System
http://macs.nu/MACS_English.pdf

FURTHER READING

Sköld A, Josephsson S, Eliasson A-C: Performing bimanual activities: the experiences of young persons with hemiplegic cerebral palsy, *Am J Occup Ther* 58:416, 2004.

22

Cleft Palate

C

Epidemiology

Cleft palate is a congenital impairment that affects one of every 600 children born in the United States. It is characterized by an opening in the roof of the mouth where the sides of the palate did not join together in utero. Cleft palate can occur unilaterally or bilaterally. Cleft palate is thought to be a result of a combination of environmental factors and genetic predisposition. Lack of folic acid has been linked to cleft palate.

Medical intervention for cleft palate includes oral surgery, which usually takes place within the child's first year of life.

Impact on Occupational Participation

- Activities of daily living
  - Eating
    - Infants with cleft palate struggle with eating because they produce inadequate suction when sucking on a nipple.

Impact on Performance Skills

- Communication and interaction skills

Impact on Client Factors (Body Functions and Structures)

- Voice and speech functions

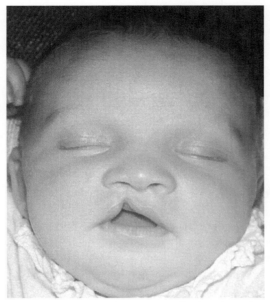

Facial view of an infant with cleft palate. (From Peterson-Falzone SJ, Hardin-Jones MA, Karnell MP: *Cleft palate speech,* ed 3, St Louis, 2001, Mosby.)

Precautions

Children with cleft palate are at greater risk for ear infections and subsequent hearing loss.

Evaluation

- Clinical observations
- Interviews with child and family
- Caregiver checklists

INTERVENTIONS

- Accommodations and modifications for feeding
- Support for the development of performance patterns related to feeding, as well as opportunities for communication

C

Case Example

Cory is a newborn infant who has been diagnosed with cleft palate. Cory's parents consult with the occupational therapist to discuss how best to position Cory during feeding and what nipple to use on his bottle. ❖

WEB RESOURCES

Cleft Palate Foundation
www.cleftline.org

Wide Smiles Cleft Lip and Palate Resource
www.widesmiles.org

FURTHER READING

Johansson B, Ringsberg K: Parents' experiences of having a child with cleft lip and palate, *J Adv Nurs* 47:165, 2004.

23

Conduct Disorder

Epidemiology

Conduct disorder is a condition found in the *Diagnostic and Statistical Manual of Mental Disorders,* 4th Edition, Text Revision (DSM-IV-TR). It affects approximately 1% to 4% of children between the ages of 9 and 17 and is more common in boys.

Children with conduct disorder engage in behavior that regularly violates age-appropriate social norms, as well as the rights of others. For children to be considered for a diagnosis of conduct disorder, this behavior must be persistent. Children age 9 and younger must demonstrate one of the following behaviors, and children age 10 and older must demonstrate three. These behaviors include the following:

- Aggression toward people and animals
- Destruction of property
- Lying, deceit, and theft
- Serious rule violations

Impact on Occupational Performance

- Social participation
- Leisure
- Work
- Education

Impact on Performance Patterns

Children with conduct disorder may demonstrate impoverished or dominating habits. In addition, they may demonstrate maladaptive routines and lack prosocial roles.

Impact on Performance Skills

- Communication and interaction skills
  - Physicality
  - Information exchange
  - Relations

Impact on Client Factors (Body Functions and Structures)

- Global mental functions
  - Temperament and personality functions
  - Energy and drive functions
- Specific mental functions
  - Thought functions
  - Emotional functions

Precautions

Children who have experienced abuse or trauma or who have attention deficit and hyperactivity disorder or other learning disabilities may be wrongly diagnosed with conduct disorder.

Evaluation

- Clinical observations
- Interviews with child and family
- Assessment tools

Suggested Assessment Tools

- Adolescent Role Assessment (ARA)
- Adolescent/Adult Sensory Profile
- Assessment of Communication and Interaction Skills (ACIS)

- Behavior Assessment Rating Scale (BASC)
- Canadian Occupational Performance Measure (COPM)
- Child and Adolescent Social Perception Measure
- Child Occupational Self Assessment (COSA)
- NIH Activity Record
- Occupational Circumstances Assessment Interview and Rating Scale (OCAIRS)
- Occupational Performance History Interview (OPHI)
- Pediatric Interest Profile (PIP)
- Perceived Efficacy and Goal Setting System (PEGS)
- Short Child Occupational Profile (SCOPE)
- Social Skills Rating System
- Test of Environmental Supportiveness
- Volitional Questionnaire (VQ)

INTERVENTIONS

- Social skill instruction
- Role exploration
- Interest exploration
- Development of useful habits and routines
- Family and caregiver training
- Self-regulation
- Prevocational skills

Case Example

John is a 15-year-old high school student who struggles with interpersonal relations. The occupational therapist provides John with social skills instruction and allows him to practice what he's learned while playing a board game in a small group of peers. ❖

WEB RESOURCES

American Academy of Child and Adolescent Psychiatry
www.aacap.org

Federation of Families for Children's Mental Health
www.ffcmh.org

FURTHER READING

Landy S, Menna R: An evaluation of group intervention for parents with aggressive young children: improvements in child functioning, maternal confidence, parenting knowledge and attitudes, *Early Child Dev Care* 176:605, 2006.

C

24

Congenital Clubfoot
(*Talipes Equinovarus*)

Epidemiology

Clubfoot is a congenital birth defect that affects approximately one in every 1000 children born in the United States. Clubfoot is characterized by the following:

- Slight shortening of the tibia
- Shortening of the fibula
- External rotation of the talus
- Medial rotation of the equinus
- Medial subluxation of the cuboid over the calcaneal head
- Adducted and supinated forefoot
- Atrophied lower extremity muscles
- Contractures in the foot and ankle
- Shortening of foot and ankle ligaments

Medical intervention for clubfoot includes casting and surgery to realign the foot and ankle. Surgery usually is performed when the child is around 6 months of age. Without medical intervention, clubfoot can result in a great deal of pain and difficulty with ambulation.

The exact cause of clubfoot is unknown.

Impact on Performance Skills

- Motor skills
  - Mobility

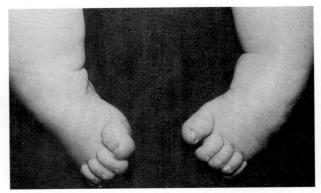

Clubfoot. (From Zitelli BJ, Davis HW: *Atlas of pediatric physical diagnosis,* ed 5, St Louis, 2007, Mosby.)

- Coordination
- Strength and effort
- Energy

Impact on Client Factors (Body Functions and Structures)
- Neuromusculoskeletal and movement-related functions
  - Functions of joints and bones
  - Muscle functions
  - Movement functions

Precautions
If left untreated, clubfoot can be very painful.

Evaluation
- Clinical observations
- Interviews with child and family
- Assessment tools

Suggested Assessment Tools
- Alberta Infant Motor Scale (AIMS)
- Bayley Scale of Infant Development (BSID)

- Denver Developmental Screening Test (DDST)
- Gross Motor Function Measure (GMFM)
- Hawaii Early Learning Profile (HELP)
- Miller Assessment for Preschoolers (MAP)
- Miller Function and Participation Scales (M-FUN-S)
- Peabody Developmental Motor Scales 2, Revised (PDMS-2)
- Pediatric Evaluation of Disability Inventory (PEDI)
- Pediatric Volitional Questionnaire (PVQ)
- Short Child Occupational Profile (SCOPE)
- Toddler and Infant Motor Evaluation (TIME)
- WeeFIM

INTERVENTIONS

- Support for the family in developing habits and routines related to medical interventions, including physical therapy
- Interventions to support play
- Interventions to support motor development
- Accommodations and modifications to the task and the environment

Case Example

Raj is a 6-month-old boy with clubfoot who receives early intervention services. Raj is undergoing casting to address clubfoot in both his lower extremities. As a result he has difficulty moving around to explore his environment. The occupational therapist works with Raj's grandmother to position him on the floor so that he can reach toys, attempt to move himself, and play. ❖

WEB RESOURCE

American Family Physician
www.aafp.org/afp/20040215/865.html

FURTHER READING

Wedge J, Daniels T, Alman B: Congenital clubfoot, *Curr Pediatr* 11:332, 2001.

25

❖

Congenital Heart Defects

Epidemiology

Congenital heart defects are a group of conditions present in newborns at birth. Approximately eight of every 1000 infants in the United States will be born with a congenital heart defect. The impact of heart defects on an infant's health and function ranges from mild to severe. A congenital heart defect implies a structural impairment of the heart that is present at birth.

Congenital heart defects are caused by a combination of genetic predisposition and environmental factors, such as maternal infections and maternal medication, and illegal drug and alcohol use. Maternal chronic illnesses also contribute to congenital heart defects.

Children with certain developmental delays (e.g., Down syndrome) are more prone to congenital heart defects.

Medical intervention for congenital heart defects includes prescription medication, surgical repair, and heart transplants.

Common congenital heart defects include the following:

- Aortic stenosis: the opening of the aortic valve is stiff and narrow and interferes with efficient pumping of the blood.
- Atrial septal defect: a hole in the wall that divides the two atria.

- Atrioventricular canal defect: rather than two valves controlling blood flow into the heart, there is only one. In addition, the central area of the heart is malformed.
- Coarctation of the aorta: a portion of the aorta is narrowed, which affects blood flow to the body.
- Hypoplastic left heart syndrome: the left side of the heart is underdeveloped.
- Patent ductus arteriosus: the ductus arteriosus blood vessel does not close on its own after birth.
- Pulmonary atresia: one pulmonary valve does not open efficiently or is missing.
- Pulmonary stenosis: the opening of the pulmonary valve is stiff and narrow and interferes with efficient pumping of the blood.
- Tetralogy of Fallot: includes pulmonary stenosis, ventricular hypertrophy, ventricular septal defect, and flow from both the right and left ventricles into the aorta.
- Total anomalous pulmonary venous connection: pulmonary vessels that are improperly joined to the left atrium.
- Transposition of the great arteries: the pulmonary artery and the aorta are switched, resulting in a decrease in oxygenated blood.
- Tricuspid atresia: the tricuspid valve is absent, and in its place is a membrane that does not allow blood flow.
- Truncus arteriosus: the pulmonary artery and aorta do not split, resulting in one common blood vessel.
- Ventricular septal defect: a hole in the wall between the two ventricles.

Signs and symptoms of congenital heart defects include bluish skin or lips, difficulty breathing, poor appetite, sweating, and decreased pulse strength.

Impact on Occupational Performance

Complications related to congenital heart defects could affect an individual's ability to participate in the following occupations:

- Activities of daily living
- Instrumental activities of daily living
- Education
- Work
- Leisure
- Social activities

Impact on Performance Patterns

Some children with congenital heart defects may experience role deprivation.

Impact on Performance Skills

Children with congenital heart defects may have typical performance skills; however, frequent hospitalizations may delay the acquisition of motor skills in some cases.

Impact on Client Factors (Body Functions and Structures)

- Cardiovascular system functions

Precautions

Congenital heart defects are serious, and some can be fatal. If a child demonstrates any of the symptoms listed previously, the emergency medical system should be alerted immediately.

Evaluation

- Clinical observations
- Interviews with child and family
- Assessment tools

Suggested Assessment Tools

- Adolescent Role Assessment (ARA)
- Assessment of Ludic Behaviors (ALB)
- Canadian Occupational Performance Measure (COPM)
- Child Behaviors Inventory of Playfulness (CBI)
- Child Occupational Self Assessment (COSA)

- Children's Assessment of Participation and Enjoyment (CAPE)
- Coping Inventory
- Knox Preschool Play Scale
- Pediatric Evaluation of Disability Inventory (PEDI)
- Pediatric Interest Profile (PIP)
- Pediatric Volitional Questionnaire (PVQ)
- Perceived Efficacy Goal Setting System (PEGS)
- Short Child Occupational Profile (SCOPE)

INTERVENTIONS

- Support for participation in all areas of occupation
- Teaching of energy conservation techniques
- Increasing of endurance through functional activities
- Child and family education about condition

Case Example

Courtney is a 3-year-old who is receiving inpatient occupational therapy after a valve replacement. Courtney fatigues easily and dislikes being in the hospital away from her friends in the neighborhood. The occupational therapist works with Courtney on increasing her endurance through participation in age-appropriate self-care and play activities. The occupational therapist also speaks with the nurse to schedule a time for her to play in the day room with other children. ❖

WEB RESOURCES

Congenital Heart Defects.com
www.congenitalheartdefects.com

March of Dimes
www.marchofdimes.com/professionals/14332_1212.asp

FURTHER READING

Mone S: Effects of environmental exposures on the cardiovascular system: prenatal period through adolescence, *Pediatrics* 113:1058, 2004.

26

❖

Congenital Obstructive Hydrocephalus

Epidemiology

Congenital obstructive hydrocephalus is a result of an obstruction of the flow of cerebrospinal fluid. It is caused by malformation of the brain structures, toxoplasmosis, and Bickers-Adams syndrome. Approximately three of every 1000 infants are born with congenital obstructive hydrocephalus.

Children with congenital obstructive hydrocephalus may complain of headaches, neck pain, and blurred or double vision. In addition, they may vomit or appear drowsy. Infants with congenital obstructive hydrocephalus may appear irritable or may be less active than usual. In addition, they may have a decreased appetite and present with vomiting. Other physical signs of congenital obstructive hydrocephalus include an enlarged head, disjunction of sutures, tense fontanelle, increased tone in the lower extremities, unsteady gait, failure to gaze upward, and sun-setting sign.

Medical intervention for congenital obstructive hydrocephalus is the surgical application of a shunt to reroute cerebrospinal fluid and lessen pressure in the skull against the brain.

Impact on Performance Skills

Congenital obstructive hydrocephalus may be accompanied by motor, process, or communication and interaction difficulties depending on the severity and whether or not the child has an associated condition.

Impact on Client Factors (Body Functions and Structures)
- Global mental functions
- Specific mental functions
- Movement-related functions

Precautions
Signs and symptoms of shunt malfunction include nausea, vomiting, and complaints of headaches. Monitor your client for these signs and symptoms, and contact emergency medical services if they persist.

Evaluation
- Clinical observations
- Interviews with child and family
- Assessment tools

Suggested Assessment Tools
- Assessment of Motor and Process Skills (AMPS)
- Canadian Occupational Performance Measure (COPM)
- Child and Adolescent Social Perception Measure
- Child Occupational Self Assessment (COSA)
- Children's Assessment of Participation and Enjoyment (CAPE)
- Dynamic Occupational Therapy Cognitive Assessment for Children (DOTCA-Ch)
- Lowenstein Occupational Therapy Cognitive Assessment (LOTCA)
- Miller Function and Participation Scales (M-FUN-S)
- Pediatric Evaluation of Disability Inventory (PEDI)
- Pediatric Interest Profile (PIP)
- Pediatric Volitional Questionnaire (PVQ)
- Perceived Efficacy and Goal Setting System (PEGS)

- School Assessment of Motor and Process Skills (School AMPS)
- School Function Assessment (SFA)
- School Setting Interview (SSI)
- Short Child Occupational Profile (SCOPE)
- WeeFIM

C

INTERVENTIONS

- Support for participation in areas of occupation
- Support for the development of motor and process skills
- Task and environmental accommodations and modifications
- Family and caregiver training and education

Case Example

Ira is a 5-month-old boy who was born at 23 weeks' gestation and has a shunt owing to congenital obstructive hydrocephalus. Ira receives early intervention occupational therapy services to address motor delays. On the last home visit, Ira's mother notes that he has been "cranky" and has had a difficult time calming down for the last 3 days. He is also taking less formula and has been spitting up. Ira's mother thinks he might be getting a cold. The occupational therapist suggests that the mother call Ira's physician immediately to see if his symptoms are related to shunt malfunction. ❖

WEB RESOURCES

Hydrocephalus Association
www.hydroassoc.org

Fetal Hydrocephalus.com
www.fetalhydrocephalus.com/hydro/default.asp

FURTHER READING

Kulkarni A: Questionnaire for assessing parents' concerns about their child with hydrocephalus, *Dev Med Child Neurol* 48:108, 2006.

27

❖

Cri Du Chat Syndrome

Epidemiology

Cri du chat syndrome is a rare genetic disorder that is a result of the deletion of a portion of the fifth chromosome. Cri du chat syndrome is sometimes referred to as *"5p– syndrome."* Children with cri du chat typically have intellectual disabilities, low birth weight, low muscle tone, and microcephaly and produce a high-pitched cry.

Nearly all children with 5p– syndrome have poor muscle tone when they are young. Other characteristics may include feeding difficulties, delays in walking, hyperactivity, scoliosis, and significant intellectual disability.

Impact on Performance Skills

- Motor skills
  - Posture
  - Mobility
  - Coordination
  - Strength and effort
- Process skills
  - Knowledge
  - Temporal organization
  - Organizing space and objects
  - Adaptation
- Communication and interaction skills
  - Physicality

- Information exchange
- Relations

Impact on Client Factors (Body Functions and Structures)

- Global mental functions
- Specific mental functions
- Voice and speech functions
- Neuromusculoskeletal and movement-related functions

Precautions

Precautions should address general safety concerns.

Evaluation

- Clinical observations
- Interviews with child and family
- Assessment tools

Suggested Assessment Tools

- Miller Function and Participation Scales (M-FUN-S)
- Pediatric Evaluation of Disability Inventory (PEDI)
- Pediatric Volitional Questionnaire (PVQ)
- School Function Assessment (SFA)
- Short Child Occupational Profile (SCOPE)

INTERVENTIONS

- Support for participation in occupations, especially activities of daily living (including toileting)
- Support for the development of fine and gross motor skills
- Support for the development of communication and interaction skills
- Support for the development of process skills
- Environmental and task accommodations and modifications

Case Example

Jordan is a 6-year-old with cri du chat. The occupational therapist is working with his mother and his teacher to develop a toileting program so that Jordan can learn to use the toilet without assistance. The occupational therapist develops a toileting schedule and a reinforcement schedule for when Jordan goes to the bathroom in the toilet. She also provides Jordan with a picture symbol and teaches him how to point to it when he is leaving to go to the bathroom. Eventually Jordan will be able to point to the picture and go to the bathroom independently. ❖

WEB RESOURCES

5p– Support Group
www.fivepminus.org

Cri Du Chat Syndrome Support Group
www.criduchat.co.uk

FURTHER READING

Campbell D, Carlin M, Justen J, Baird SM: *Cru-du-chat syndrome: a topical overview*, 2004. Available at: www.fivepminus.org/cdc%20overview.pdf. Accessed May 13, 2007.

28

Cystic Fibrosis

Epidemiology

Cystic fibrosis (CF) is a recessive genetic condition (chromosome 7) that affects an individual's lungs, pancreas, liver, intestines, sinuses, and reproductive organs. Individuals with CF may have presentations that are quite different. Some children are likely to experience serious challenges from birth on, whereas others may not have complications related to CF until adolescence or young adulthood.

Approximately 30,000 individuals in the United States have CF. CF is a life-threatening condition. Life expectancy for individuals with CF averages 36.5 years.

Impact on Performance Patterns

Some children with cystic fibrosis may experience role deprivation owing to frequent hospitalizations. Children will also have to develop supportive habits related to their medical interventions.

Impact on Performance Skills

Individuals may not experience a delay in the development of motor, process, or communication and interaction skills.

Impact on Client Factors (Body Functions and Structures)

- Respiratory system functions
- Digestive system functions
- Reproductive system functions

Precautions

Individuals with CF are at greater risk for respiratory infections.

Evaluation

- Clinical observations
- Interviews with child and family
- Assessment tools

Suggested Assessment Tools

- Pediatric Interest Profile (PIP)
- Canadian Occupational Performance Measure (COPM)
- Pediatric Activity Card Sort (PACS)
- Child Occupational Self Assessment (COSA)
- Perceived Efficacy and Goal Setting System (PEGS)
- School Setting Interview (SSI)
- Short Child Occupational Profile (SCOPE)

INTERVENTIONS

- Interest exploration
- Role exploration
- Support for the development of habits and routines related to medication management
- Education of child about signs and symptoms of an exacerbation
- Environmental modifications (e.g., reduction of irritants)
- School accommodations
- Leisure-related accommodations and modifications

Case Example

Becky is a seventh-grade student with CF. Becky does not receive special education services at school, but she does have a 504 plan to provide her with educationally related accommodations and modifications. The occupational therapist was instrumental in helping the school team develop a plan to meet Becky's needs. Some of her accommodations include allowing a classmate to copy down homework assignments and share them with her when she is out of the room taking her medication, providing her with audiotaped lessons for days of school that she misses, and allowing her extra time on long-range assignments if she is absent between the time they are assigned and their due dates. ❖

WEB RESOURCES

Cystic Fibrosis Foundation
www.cff.org

March of Dimes
www.marchofdimes.com/pnhec/4439_1213.asp

FURTHER READING

Gayer D, Ganong L: Family structure and mothers' caregiving of children with cystic fibrosis, *J Fam Nurs* 12:390, 2006.

29

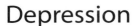

Depression

Epidemiology

It is estimated that approximately 1% to 3% of young children and 3% to 9% of adolescents meet the diagnostic criteria for depression as it is classified in the *Diagnostic and Statistical Manual of Mental Disorders,* 4th Edition, Text Revision (DSM-IV-TR). Depression is thought to be caused by a combination of genetic factors and stressful events that leads to an imbalance of neurotransmitters. In addition, some medications, as well as other medical conditions, can trigger depression.

Signs and symptoms of depression include a state of persistent sadness, hopelessness, increased irritability or agitation, a tendency to withdraw from friends, altered sleeping and eating patterns, indecisiveness, decreased attention, decreased self-efficacy, increased complaints of physical pain, low energy, drug or alcohol use, and suicidal ideation.

Impact on Performance Skills
- Knowledge
  - Chooses
  - Uses
  - Handles
  - Heeds
  - Inquires

- Temporal organization
  - Initiates
  - Continues
  - Sequences
  - Terminates
- Organization of space and objects
  - Searches and locates
  - Gathers
  - Organizes
  - Restores
  - Navigates
- Adaptation
  - Notices and responds
  - Accommodates
  - Adjusts
- Physicality
  - Contacts
  - Maneuvers
- Information exchange
  - Expresses
  - Modulates
- Relations
  - Collaborates
  - Conforms
  - Focuses
  - Relates
  - Respects

Impact on Client Factors (Body Functions and Structures)

- Global mental functions
  - Sleep
  - Temperament and personality functions
  - Energy and drive functions
- Specific mental functions
  - Attention functions

- Memory functions
- Thought functions

Precautions

Any child who discusses or otherwise indicates suicidal thoughts or behaviors should be taken seriously. Children with bipolar disorder are also at risk for engaging in dangerous or risky behavior.

D

Evaluation

- Clinical observations
- Interviews with child and family
- Assessment tools

Suggested Assessment Tools

- Assessment of Motor and Process Skills (AMPS)
- Canadian Occupational Performance Measure (COPM)
- Child and Adolescent Social Perception Measure
- Child Occupational Self Assessment (COSA)
- Dynamic Occupational Therapy Cognitive Assessment for Children (DOTCA-Ch)
- Lowenstein Occupational Therapy Cognitive Assessment (LOTCA)
- Miller Function and Participation Scales (M-FUN-S)
- Pediatric Volitional Questionnaire (PVQ)
- Perceived Efficacy and Goal Setting System (PEGS)
- School Assessment of Motor and Process Skills (School AMPS)
- School Function Assessment (SFA)
- School Setting Interview (SSI)
- Short Child Occupational Profile (SCOPE)
- Social Skills Rating System
- Test of Everyday Attention for Children (TEA-Ch)

INTERVENTIONS

- Support for the development of habits and routines
- Support for coping with and reducing stressors
- Environmental accommodations and modifications
- Cognitive behavioral therapy and metacognitive strategies leading to self-regulation (e.g., self-monitoring and self-evaluation)
- Teaching of relaxation techniques
- Addressing of occupational performance in activities of daily living, IADLS, education, play, leisure, and social and community participation
- Family and caregiver training and education
- Role exploration
- Prevocational skills training

Case Example

Kevin is a 14-year-old boy who has been diagnosed with bipolar disorder. Kevin struggles with getting out of bed in the morning and coming to school. The occupational therapist works with him to use metacognitive strategies related to self-regulation, such as goal setting, self-monitoring, and self-evaluation to help him develop supportive habits so that he can get to school on time. ❖

WEB RESOURCES

National Alliance on Mental Illness
www.nami.org

Mental Health Research Association
www.narsad.org/dc/depression

FURTHER READING

Compton S, March J, Brent D, et al: Cognitive-behavioral psychotherapy for anxiety and depressive disorders in children and adolescents: An evidence-based medicine review, *J Am Acad Child Adolesc Psychiatry* 43:930, 2004.

30

Developmental Coordination Disorder

Epidemiology

Children with developmental coordination disorder (DCD) demonstrate impaired motor coordination. It is estimated that approximately 6% of children aged 5 to 11 years have DCD.

Symptoms of DCD include delays in meeting motor milestones, as well as gross and fine motor clumsiness or incoordination. The cause of DCD is unknown.

Impact on Performance Skills

- Motor skills
  - Coordination
    - Coordinates
    - Manipulates
    - Flows

Impact on Client Factors (Body Functions and Structures)

- Motor functions

Precautions

Children with DCD are at risk for difficulties related to decreased volition, such as low academic performance, poor self-esteem, and infrequent physical activity. In addition, they may incur frequent injuries as a result of their incoordination.

Evaluation
- Clinical observations
- Interviews with child and family
- Assessment tools

D

Suggested Assessment Tools
- Assessment of Motor and Process Skills (AMPS)
- Bruininks-Oseretsky Test of Motor Performance (BOT-2)
- Beery-Butenica Developmental Test of Visual Motor Integration (VMI)
- Benton Constructional Praxis Test
- Canadian Occupational Performance Measure (COPM)
- Child Occupational Self Assessment (COSA)
- Children's Assessment of Participation and Enjoyment (CAPE)
- Children's Handwriting Evaluation Scale (CHES)
- Evaluation Tool of Children's Handwriting (ETCH)
- Gross Motor Function Measure (GMFM)
- Lincoln-Oseretsky Motor Development Scale
- Miller Function and Participation Scales (M-FUN-S)
- Movement Assessment Battery for Children (Movement ABC)
- Peabody Developmental Motor Scales 2, Revised (PDMS-2)
- Pediatric Activity Card Sort (PACS)
- Perceived Efficacy and Goal Setting System (PEGS)
- School Function Assessment (SFA)
- School Setting Interview (SSI)
- Short Child Occupational Profile (SCOPE)

INTERVENTIONS

- Support for motor development leading to increased participation in occupations
- Teaching of metacognitive strategies to develop motor plans
- Support for problem solving for execution of motor plans
- Suggestions for accommodations and modifications to tasks and environments

D

Case Example

Charlie is an 8-year-old boy with DCD who has trouble getting dressed in the morning. Despite practice, Charlie continues to struggle with buttoning and shoe-tying. Charlie wants to get dressed himself. The occupational therapist works with Charlie to find clothing, such as pullover tops and pants without buttons, that he can put on himself when he is trying to get dressed quickly for school. In addition, the occupational therapist works with Charlie to develop strategies to complete other motor tasks, such as neatly putting away laundry and playing basketball. ❖

WEB RESOURCES

CanChild Centre for Childhood Disability Research
www.canchild.ca/Default.aspx?tabid=468

Dyspraxia USA NFP
www.dyspraxiausa.org/About_Us.html

FURTHER READING

Bernie C, Rodger S: Cognitive strategy use in school-aged children with developmental coordination disorder, *Phys Occup Ther Pediatr* 24:23, 2004.

31

❖

Disseminated Intravascular Coagulation

Epidemiology

Disseminated intravascular coagulation (DIC) is a secondary medical condition that can result from many factors, including but not limited to infections, complications in pregnancy, cancer, burns, and severe trauma. DIC prevents an individual's blood from clotting normally and can lead to the formation of thrombosis or hemorrhaging, which can ultimately result in death.

DIC is usually diagnosed through laboratory tests and is treated medically by removal of the cause if possible, transfusions, and medication. On some occasions an individual may demonstrate signs and symptoms before diagnosis. These include bruising, small red dots under the skin, heavy bleeding from the mouth or nose, shortness of breath, and low blood pressure.

Impact on Performance Skills

DIC is an acute medical condition that will likely affect all performance skills temporarily.

Impact on Client Factors (Body Functions and Structures)

• Hematologic system functions
• Possible impact on other organ system functions

Precautions

DIC is usually seen as a secondary condition. Because DIC prevents an individual's blood from clotting normally, this condition can lead to death.

Evaluation

- Clinical observations
- Interviews with child and family
- Assessment tools

Suggested Assessment Tools

Because DIC is a secondary condition, the occupational therapist should choose assessment tools based on the primary condition.

INTERVENTION

- Interventions will be based on the primary condition.

WEB RESOURCE

Centers for Disease Control and Prevention
www.bt.cdc.gov/training/smallpoxvaccine/reactions/septicshock2.html

FURTHER READING

Barret J, Gomez P: Disseminated intravascular coagulation: a rare entity in burn injury, *Burns* 31:354, 2005.

32

❖

Down Syndrome
(Trisomy 21)

Epidemiology

Down syndrome (DS) is a genetic condition that is caused by three copies of the twenty-first chromosome. DS occurs in approximately one in 800 to 1000 infants. Most individuals with DS share common characteristics, which include intellectual disability and facial features. In addition, it is estimated that 30% to 50% of individuals with DS may also have heart defects, and 8% to 12% experience gastrointestinal malformations.

Individuals with DS have unique characteristics, which include the following:

- Upward-slanting palpebral fissures
- Flat nasal bridge
- Epicanthal folds
- Smaller, shorter fingers and shorter hands
- Fewer bones
- Lower-set thumb
- Small or missing middle phalanx on the fifth digits
- Hypotonia
- Absence of palmar creases
- Poorly formed skin patterns, which affects sensation

Children with DS are also more likely to experience other health problems, including the following:

D

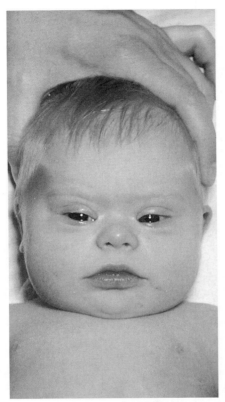

Down syndrome. (From Zitelli BJ, Davis HW: *Atlas of pediatric physical diagnosis*, ed 5, St Louis, 2007, Mosby.)

- Intellectual disability
- Heart defects
- Intestinal defects
- Vision problems
- Hearing loss
- Memory loss

Impact on Performance Skills

- Motor skills
  - Posture
  - Mobility
  - Coordination
  - Strength and effort
  - Energy
- Process skills
  - Energy
  - Knowledge
  - Temporal organization
  - Organizing space and objects
  - Adaptation
- Communication and interaction skills
  - Information exchange

Impact on Client Factors (Body Functions and Structures)

- Global mental functions
- Specific mental functions
- Sensory functions (hearing, vision, and touch functions)
- Muscle functions
- Movement functions
- Cardiovascular system functions
- Digestive system functions

Precautions

Approximately 10% to 30% of individuals with DS have a condition called *atlantoaxial instability* (AAI), which is caused by abnormalities of ligaments that maintain the atlantoaxial joint. AAI is dangerous because it can lead to permanent neurologic damage from spinal cord compression. Individuals with AAI should never do somersaults and should receive medical clearance for all sports.

Evaluation
- Clinical observations
- Interviews with child and family
- Assessment tools

Suggested Assessment Tools
- Alberta Infant Motor Scale (AIMS)
- Assessment of Motor and Process Skills (AMPS)
- Bayley Scale of Infant Development (BSID)
- Beery-Butenica Developmental Test of Visual Motor Integration (VMI)
- Benton Constructional Praxis Test
- Canadian Occupational Performance Measure (COPM)
- Child Occupational Self Assessment (COSA)
- Children's Assessment of Participation and Enjoyment (CAPE)
- Children's Handwriting Evaluation Scale (CHES)
- Denver Developmental Screening Test (DDST)
- Evaluation Tool of Children's Handwriting (ETCH)
- Gross Motor Function Measure (GMFM)
- Hawaii Early Learning Profile (HELP)
- Lincoln-Oseretsky Motor Development Scale
- Miller Function and Participation Scales (M-FUN-S)
- Movement Assessment Battery for Children (Movement ABC)
- Peabody Developmental Motor Scales 2, Revised (PDMS-2)
- Pediatric Activity Card Sort (PACS)
- Pediatric Evaluation of Disability Inventory (PEDI)
- Perceived Efficacy and Goal Setting System (PEGS)
- School Function Assessment (SFA)
- School Setting Interview (SSI)
- Short Child Occupational Profile (SCOPE)
- Toddler and Infant Motor Evaluation (TIME)
- Vineland Adaptive Behavior Scale (VABS)
- WeeFIM

INTERVENTIONS

- Activities of daily living
- Instrumental activities of daily living
- Education
- Leisure
- Prevocational skills training
- Accommodations and modifications
- Support for the development of muscle strength and motor coordination
- Support for the development of process skills
- Support for the development of motor and communication and interaction skills
- Environment and task accommodations and modifications
- Family coaching and training
- Support for the development of self-determination skills

D

Case Example

Connie is a 4-year-old girl with DS who attends a half-day early childhood program. The occupational therapist works with Connie on increasing fine motor strength and coordination so that she can complete art projects and play at various centers with her peers. ❖

WEB RESOURCES

National Down Syndrome Society
www.ndss.org

National Association for Down Syndrome
www.nads.org

FURTHER READING

Edwards S: Hand function of children with Down's syndrome, *Dev Disabil Spec Interest Sect Q AOTA* 21:1, 1998.

33

❖

Dysrhythmias

Epidemiology

Dysrhythmias, also called *arrhythmias* or *abnormal heart rates,* are characterized by atypical heart rhythms such as tachycardia or bradycardia. Dysrhythmia occurs when the electrical impulse that regulates the contraction of the heart happens too quickly or too slowly or skips beats.

Dysrhythmia may be caused by heart conditions, endocrine imbalances, and drug use.

Symptoms of dysrhythmia include the following:
- Quick or slow heart beats
- Skipped heart beats
- Dizziness
- Shortness of breath
- Fainting
- Chest pain
- Sweating
- Cardiac arrest

Impact on Performance Skills

Dysrhythmia is an acute medical condition that will likely affect all performance skills temporarily.

Impact on Client Factors (Body Functions and Structures)

- Cardiovascular functions

Precautions

Dysrhythmia is associated with cardiac arrest. Individuals with dysrhythmia should be monitored during therapeutic activities.

Evaluation

- Clinical observations
- Interviews with child and family
- Assessment tools

Suggested Assessment Tools

Dysrhythmia may not be the primary reason for the occupational therapy referral. Assessment tools should address the primary reason for referral.

INTERVENTION

- Intervention should address the primary reason for referral.

WEB RESOURCES

UCSF Pediatric Arrhythmia Center
www.ucsfhealth.org/childrens/medical_services/heart_center/ arrhythmia/index.htm

Cardiac Arrhythmias Research and Education Center
www.longqt.org

FURTHER READING

Rosenberg D, Moss M: Guidelines and levels of care for pediatric intensive care units, *Pediatrics* 114:1114, 2004.

34

❖

Edwards' Syndrome (Trisomy 18)

Epidemiology

Edwards' syndrome, or trisomy 18, is a genetic condition that is caused by three copies of the eighteenth chromosome. Edwards' syndrome occurs in approximately one in 3000 to 5000 infants. It is different from other trisomies because it is usually fatal. Most babies born with Edwards' syndrome typically live only a few days, with a small percentage living 1 year.

Individuals with Edwards' syndrome share unique characteristics, which include the following:

- Small head size
- Prominence of the back part of the head
- Short eyelid fissures
- Small mouth and jaw
- Small fingernails
- Underdeveloped or altered thumbs
- Short sternum

In addition, individuals born with Edwards' syndrome are often born with other medical conditions, such as the following:

- Club foot
- Congenital heart defects
- Joint contractures

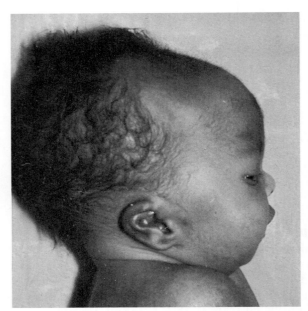

Physical manifestations of trisomy 18. A typical profile reveals prominent occiput and low-set, posteriorly rotated malformed auricles. (From Zitelli BJ, Davis HW: *Atlas of pediatric physical diagnosis,* ed 5, St Louis, 2007, Mosby.)

- Hearing loss
- Cleft lip
- Spina bifida
- Radial aplasia
- Micrognathia
- Esophageal atresia
- Kidney abnormalities
- Omphalocele

Impact on Performance Skills

- Motor skills
- Process skills
- Communication and interaction skills

Impact on Client Factors (Body Functions and Structures)

- Mental functions
- Sensory functions
- Neuromusculoskeletal functions
- Cardiovascular functions
- Digestive and metabolic functions

Precautions

Because of the numerous associated conditions, children with Edwards' syndrome are likely to have numerous precautions and to be classified as "medically fragile." Therapists should be sure to know the family's wishes about resuscitation.

Evaluation

- Clinical observations
- Interviews with family

INTERVENTIONS

- Provision of support and education to families and caregivers
- Positioning
- Feeding if able
- Environmental modifications to reduce noxious sensory input in the neonatal intensive care unit (NICU)

Case Example

The occupational therapist is working in the NICU with Joey, a premature infant who was born with Edwards' syndrome, and his parents. Joey's mother and father understand the seriousness of Joey's condition and are afraid to pick him up or interact with in almost any way. The occupational therapist works with them to read Joey's cues and instructs them on how to hold him for short periods throughout the day. ✧

WEB RESOURCES

Trisomy 18 Foundation
www.trisomy18.org

Support Organization for Trisomy 18, 13 and Related Disorders (SOFT)
www.trisomy.org

FURTHER READING

Romesberg T: Understanding grief: a component of neonatal palliative care, *J Hosp Palliat Nurs* 6:161, 2004.

35

❖

Epilepsy (Seizure Disorder)

Epidemiology

Epilepsy, or seizure disorder, is a neurologic condition that affects approximately eight of every 1000 people. Epilepsy is characterized by transient but recurrent seizures. A seizure is an unexpected, excessive discharge of electrical activity in the brain that alters the individual's behavior temporarily. Premature infants and those who are born with abnormal brain structures or have been deprived of oxygen are at greater risk for developing seizures. Family history of seizures, high fevers, and acquired brain injuries also increase the risk for seizures.

Individuals may experience seizures differently. For example, some individuals may lose consciousness, whereas others may only look "spaced out." Some individuals may demonstrate physical characteristics, such as chewing movements, convulsions, difficulty talking, drooling, eye movements, foot stomping, shaking, staring, sweating, difficulty breathing, and tremors.

After an individual has a seizure, he or she may experience memory loss or confusion. In addition, that person may be very sleepy and feel weak.

Impact on Performance Skills

- Motor skills may be temporarily affected.
- Process skills may be temporarily affected.

- Communication and interaction skills may be temporarily affected.

Impact on Client Factors (Body Functions and Structures)

- Global mental functions may be temporarily affected.
- Specific mental functions may be temporarily affected.
- Structures of the nervous system.

Precautions

Warning signs of seizures include vision loss or blurring, reports of "feeling strange," dizziness, headache, lightheadedness, and nausea. Children who are having seizures should not be left alone. Those who have physical seizures should be placed in a side-lying position, and the head should be protected if the child is having convulsions. If an individual vomits while having a seizure, be sure to clear his or her airway. Prolonged seizures should be treated as medical emergencies.

Evaluation

Occupational therapy evaluation will likely be for conditions associated with epilepsy, such as acquired brain injury or cerebral palsy.

INTERVENTION

Occupational therapy intervention will likely be necessary for conditions associated with epilepsy, such as acquired brain injury or cerebral palsy.

WEB RESOURCES

Epilepsy.com
www.epilepsy.com

Epilepsy Foundation
www.epilepsyfoundation.org

FURTHER READING

Vestergaard M, Pedersen C, Sidenius P, et al: The long-term risk of epilepsy after febrile seizures in susceptible subgroups, *Am J Epidemiol* 165:911, 2007.

E

36

❖

Fetal Alcohol Syndrome Disorders

Epidemiology

Fetal alcohol syndrome disorders (FASDs) consist of three conditions that are caused by prenatal alcohol exposure: fetal alcohol effects (FAE), alcohol-related neurodevelopmental disorder (ARND), and alcohol-related birth defects (ARBD). FASDs are characterized by abnormal facial features, growth deficiencies, intellectual disabilities, and central nervous systems problems. In addition, some children may have behavioral disabilities. FASDs are estimated to affect 1.5 to 4.5 of every 1000 live births and are totally preventable. FASDs occur because alcohol in the mother's blood crosses the placenta and enters the embryo or fetus through the umbilical cord. Drinking alcohol at any time during pregnancy can have adverse effects on fetal development.

Common characteristics of FASDs include the following:
- Small stature compared with same age peers
- Facial abnormalities
- Poor coordination
- Hyperactivity
- Learning or intellectual disabilities
- Delays in development
- Sleeping and eating disturbances

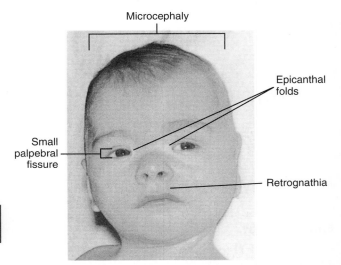

Fetal alcohol syndrome. (From Thibodeau GA, Patton KT: *Anatomy and physiology,* ed 6, St Louis, 2007, Mosby.)

Impact on Performance Skills

- Motor skills
  - Coordinates
  - Manipulates
  - Flows
- Process skills
  - Paces
  - Attends
  - Chooses
  - Handles
  - Uses
  - Heeds
  - Inquires
  - Initiates
  - Continues
  - Sequences
  - Terminates

- Organizes space and objects
- Adapts to environmental demands

Impact on Client Factors (Body Functions and Structures)
- Global mental functions
- Specific mental functions

Precautions
No precautions have been noted.

Evaluation
- Clinical observations
- Interviews with child and family
- Assessment tools

Suggested Assessment Tools
- Alberta Infant Motor Scale (AIMS)
- Assessment of Motor and Process Skills (AMPS)
- Bayley Scale of Infant Development (BSID)
- Beery-Butenica Developmental Test of Visual Motor Integration (VMI)
- Canadian Occupational Performance Measure (COPM)
- Children's Assessment of Participation and Enjoyment (CAPE)
- Children's Handwriting Evaluation Scale (CHES)
- Evaluation Tool of Children's Handwriting (ETCH)
- Gross Motor Function Measure (GMFM)
- Hawaii Early Learning Profile (HELP)
- Lincoln-Oseretsky Motor Development Scale
- Miller Function and Participation Scales (M-FUN-S)
- Movement Assessment Battery for Children (Movement ABC)
- Peabody Developmental Motor Scales 2, Revised (PDMS-2)
- Pediatric Activity Card Sort (PACS)
- Pediatric Evaluation of Disability Inventory (PEDI)
- Pediatric Volitional Questionnaire (PVQ)

- Perceived Efficacy and Goal Setting System (PEGS)
- School Function Assessment (SFA)
- Short Child Occupational Profile (SCOPE)
- Social Skills Rating System
- Test of Everyday Attention for Children (TEA-Ch)
- Toddler and Infant Motor Evaluation (TIME)
- WeeFIM

INTERVENTIONS

- Support for participation and independence in activities of daily living
- Support for participation and independence in instrumental activities of daily living
- Support for the development of motor and process skills
- Support for participation and independence at school
- Task and environmental accommodations and modifications

Case Example

Charmaine is a 4-year-old girl with FASD who lives in foster care and attends early childhood special education. Charmaine has delayed fine motor coordination skills and mild intellectual disabilities. The occupational therapist works with Charmaine on cutting, coloring, and completing routine circle time activities. ❖

WEB RESOURCES

Fetal Alcohol Disorders and Society
www.faslink.org

National Organization on Fetal Alcohol Syndrome
www.nofas.org

FURTHER READING

Schonfeld A, Paley B, Frankel F, O'Connor MJ: Executive functioning predicts social skills following prenatal alcohol exposure, *Child Neuropsychol* 12:439, 2006.

37

❖

Fragile X Syndrome

Epidemiology

Fragile X syndrome (FXS) affects approximately one in 4000 males and one in 6000 females. FXS is the most common inherited cause of intellectual disabilities and developmental delays. FXS is caused by a mutation on the *FMR1* or *FMR2* gene on the X chromosome that is needed for normal brain development.

Children with FXS develop characteristic facial features as they get older. These facial features include the following:

- Large head
- Long face
- Prominent ears, chin, and forehead

FXS is diagnosed through a DNA sample.

Impact on Performance Skills

- Motor skills
  - Posture
  - Mobility
  - Coordination
  - Strength and effort
  - Energy
- Process skills
  - Energy
  - Knowledge

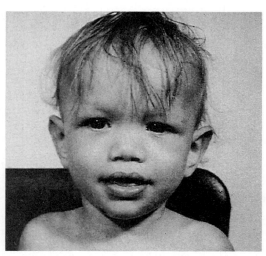

Fragile X syndrome. Note the long, wide, and protruding ears, elongated face, and flattened nasal bridge. (From Simko A, Hornstein L, Soukup S, Bagamery N: Fragile X syndrome: recognition in young children, *Pediatrics* 83:547, 1989.)

- Temporal organization
- Organization of space and objects
- Adaptation
- Communication and interaction skills
  - Information exchange

Impact on Client Factors (Body Functions and Structures)

- Global mental functions
- Specific mental functions
- Sensory functions

Precautions

No precautions have been noted.

Evaluation
- Clinical observations
- Interviews with child and family
- Assessment tools

Suggested Assessment Tools
- Alberta Infant Motor Scale (AIMS)
- Assessment of Motor and Process Skills (AMPS)
- Bayley Scale of Infant Development (BSID)
- Beery-Butenica Developmental Test of Visual Motor Integration (VMI)
- Canadian Occupational Performance Measure (COPM)
- Child Occupational Self Assessment (COSA)
- Children's Assessment of Participation and Enjoyment (CAPE)
- Children's Handwriting Evaluation Scale (CHES)
- Denver Developmental Screening Test (DDST)
- Evaluation Tool of Children's Handwriting (ETCH)
- Gross Motor Function Measure (GMFM)
- Hawaii Early Learning Profile (HELP)
- Infant/Toddler Sensory Profile
- Lincoln-Oseretsky Motor Development Scale
- Miller Function and Participation Scales (M-FUN-S)
- Movement Assessment Battery for Children (Movement ABC)
- Peabody Developmental Motor Scales 2, Revised (PDMS-2)
- Pediatric Activity Card Sort (PACS)
- Pediatric Evaluation of Disability Inventory (PEDI)
- Perceived Efficacy and Goal Setting System (PEGS)
- School Function Assessment (SFA)
- Sensory Processing Measure (SPM)
- Sensory Profile
- Short Child Occupational Profile (SCOPE)
- Toddler and Infant Motor Evaluation (TIME)
- Vineland Adaptive Behavior Scale (VABS)
- WeeFIM

INTERVENTIONS

- Activities of daily living
- Instrumental activities of daily living
- Education
- Leisure
- Prevocational skills training
- Accommodations and modifications
- Support for the development of muscle strength and motor coordination
- Support for the development of process skills
- Support for the development of motor and communication and interaction skills
- Environment and task accommodations and modifications
- Family coaching and training
- Support for the development of self-determination skills

Case Example

Saul is a 14-year-old with FXS who would eventually like to work at the local hardware store in his community. The occupational therapist works with Saul's Individualized Education Plan team to develop transition goals related to applying for jobs and interview skills. ❖

WEB RESOURCES

National Fragile X Foundation
www.fragilex.org/html/testing.htm

March of Dimes
www.marchofdimes.com/pnhec/4439_9266.asp

FURTHER READING

Baranek G, Chin Y, Hess L, et al: Sensory processing correlates of occupational performance in children with fragile X syndrome: preliminary findings, *Am J Occup Ther* 56:538, 2002.

38

❖

Galactosemia

Epidemiology

Galactosemia is a genetic disease that results in a lack of a liver enzyme required to digest galactose, which is commonly found in dairy products. Galactosemia is not usually noticeable at birth; however, shortly thereafter the infant fails to gain weight and experiences diarrhea, jaundice, and vomiting.

For unknown reasons some children with galactosemia may develop speech delays, fine and gross motor incoordination, or learning disabilities as they get older. Cataracts are another possible complication of galactosemia.

Impact on Performance Skills
- Motor skills
  - Mobility
  - Coordination
  - Strength and effort
- Process skills
  - Energy
  - Knowledge
  - Temporal organization
  - Organization of space and objects
  - Adaptation
- Communication and interaction skills
  - Information exchange

Impact on Client Factors (Body Functions and Structures)

- Digestive functions
- Metabolic functions
- Movement functions
- Speech functions
- Specific mental functions

Precautions

Galactosemia is a serious condition. If it is not detected immediately, infants are at risk for serious infections, liver disease, cataracts, intellectual disabilities, and even death. The American Liver Foundation recommends that all infants who develop jaundice be evaluated for galactosemia. If an infant ingested galactose, through formula or breast milk, he or she can develop sepsis and will usually be given a course of antibiotics. Even after an infant has been switched to a soy-based formula, sepsis may still develop if the infant ingested galactose in the past.

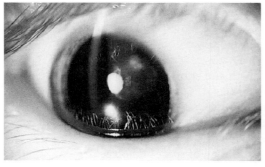

Cataract of galactosemia. (From Zitelli BJ, Davis HW: *Atlas of pediatric physical diagnosis,* ed 5, St Louis, 2007, Mosby.)

Evaluation
- Clinical observations
- Interviews with child and family
- Assessment tools

Suggested Assessment Tools
- Alberta Infant Motor Scale (AIMS)
- Assessment of Motor and Process Skills (AMPS)
- Bayley Scale of Infant Development (BSID)
- Beery-Butenica Developmental Test of Visual Motor Integration (VMI)
- Benton Constructional Praxis Test
- Canadian Occupational Performance Measure (COPM)
- Child Occupational Self Assessment (COSA)
- Children's Assessment of Participation and Enjoyment (CAPE)
- Children's Handwriting Evaluation Scale (CHES)
- Denver Developmental Screening Test (DDST)
- Evaluation Tool of Children's Handwriting (ETCH)
- Gross Motor Function Measure (GMFM)
- Hawaii Early Learning Profile (HELP)
- Lincoln-Oseretsky Motor Development Scale
- Miller Function and Participation Scales (M-FUN-S)
- Movement Assessment Battery for Children (Movement ABC)
- Peabody Developmental Motor Scales 2, Revised (PDMS-2)
- Pediatric Activity Card Sort (PACS)
- Pediatric Evaluation of Disability Inventory (PEDI)
- Perceived Efficacy and Goal Setting System (PEGS)
- School Function Assessment (SFA)
- School Setting Interview (SSI)
- Short Child Occupational Profile (SCOPE)
- Toddler and Infant Motor Evaluation (TIME)
- WeeFIM

G

INTERVENTIONS

- Activities of daily living
- Instrumental activities of daily living
- Education
- Leisure
- Prevocational skills training
- Accommodations and modifications
- Support for the development of process skills
- Support for the development of motor and communication and interaction skills
- Environment and task accommodations and modifications

G

Case Example

Regina is a 15-year-old with galactosemia and a mild intellectual disability. Regina attends an extracurricular cooking class at her community park district. Regina's physician provided her with a list of foods and beverages to which she is allergic. Although all the staff members are aware of her allergies, Regina wants to be able to read food labels and make choices about what she can and cannot eat or drink. The occupational therapist works with Regina to locate ingredients on food labels and find ingredients to which she is allergic by matching the words on the label with a preprinted list of her allergies. ❖

WEB RESOURCE

Parents of Galactosemic Children
www.galactosemia.org

FURTHER READING

Garden A, Davidson D: Recommendations for the management of galactosemia, *Arch Dis Child* 82:266, 2000.

39

❖

Gastroschisis

Epidemiology

Gastroschisis is a birth defect characterized by a hernia in which an infant's intestines protrude out of the body through a hole in the abdominal wall, typically on the right side of the umbilical cord. This condition may be detected during fetal ultrasound or apparent at birth during delivery.

Gut motility and absorption are affected owing to the unprotected intestine being exposed to irritating amniotic fluid in utero.

Medical intervention includes surgery within the first few weeks of life to put the intestine back in the abdomen and close the defect.

Impact on Occupational Participation
- Activities of daily living
  - Feeding

Impact on Client Factors (Body Functions and Structures)
- Digestive system functions

Precautions

Before surgery the infant's temperature must be closely monitored, as body heat may escape from the exposed intestine.

Infants may also have difficulty with feeding or may experience gastroesophageal reflux.

Evaluation
- Clinical observations
- Chart review
- Interviews with child and medical staff

INTERVENTIONS
- Family and caregiver training and education
- Intervention for feeding

Case Example

Nikki is a 2-day-old infant with gastroschisis in the neonatal intensive care unit. The occupational therapist educates her family about her condition and discusses precautions related to maintaining her temperature. ❖

WEB RESOURCE
www.nlm.nih.gov/medlineplus/ency/article/000992.htm

FURTHER READING
Glasser J: Omphalocele and gastroschisis, 2006. Available at: *www.emedicine. com/ped/topic1642.htm*. Accessed May 17, 2007.

40

❖

Hemophilia

Epidemiology

Hemophilia is a blood disorder usually affecting males in which one of the proteins that is needed to clot the blood is missing or reduced. This leads to longer bleeding times, which are called *bleeding episodes*. Approximately 60% of the cases of hemophilia can be traced back to hereditary causes. Depending on the severity of the condition, joint mobility may be affected.

There are three different types of hemophilia:

- Mild hemophilia: bleeding episodes are usually seen after serious injuries or trauma. Hemophilia is not usually detected until such an incident occurs.
- Moderate hemophilia: bleeding episodes tend to occur after minor injuries or without obvious cause.
- Severe hemophilia: bleeding episodes occur after injuries or without obvious cause and may affect joints and muscles.

Signs and symptoms of hemophilia include the following:

- Excessive bleeding
- Excessive bruising
- Spontaneous bleeding or bleeding with no obvious known cause
- Nosebleeds

H

Impact on Performance Skills
- Motor skills
  - Mobility
  - Coordination
  - Strength and effort
- Process skills
  - Energy
  - Knowledge
  - Temporal organization
  - Organization of space and objects
  - Adaptation
- Communication and interaction skills
  - Information exchange

Impact on Client Factors (Body Functions and Structures)
- Digestive functions
- Metabolic functions
- Movement functions
- Speech functions
- Specific mental functions

Precautions
Children who receive small cuts should be treated with first aid. Individuals with mild hemophilia may use a product called *desmopressin acetate* (DDAVP) to treat small bleeds; however, deeper cuts will require medical treatment.

Evaluation
- Clinical observations
- Interviews with child and family
- Range of motion
- Assessment tools

Suggested Assessment Tools
- Assessment of Motor and Process Skills (AMPS)
- Bruininks-Oseretsky Test of Motor Performance (BOT-2)

- Canadian Occupational Performance Measure (COPM)
- Child Occupational Self Assessment (COSA)
- Gross Motor Function Measure (GMFM)
- Lincoln-Oseretsky Motor Development Scale
- Miller Function and Participation Scales (M-FUN-S)
- Movement Assessment Battery for Children (Movement ABC)
- Perceived Efficacy and Goal Setting System (PEGS)
- Short Child Occupational Profile (SCOPE)

INTERVENTIONS

- Activities and exercises to maintain joint range of motion
- Accommodations and modifications
- Support for the child's medication management
- Support for participation in activities of daily living
- Promotion of problem solving and safety awareness

H

Case Example

Brian is a 16-year-old who is receiving occupational therapy out-patient rehabilitation services because of a mild acquired brain injury that he sustained as a result of a motor vehicle accident. In addition to his acquired brain injury, Brian also has hemophilia. The occupational therapist is working with Brian on sequencing during a grooming activity. In addition to working on sequencing, the occupational therapist is also working with him on problem solving and safety awareness. The occupational therapist talks with Brian about what he would do if he happened to cut himself while shaving. ❖

WEB RESOURCES

National Hemophilia Foundation
www.hemophilia.org

Hemophilia Federation of America
www.hemophiliafed.org

FURTHER READING

Gurcay E, Eksioglu E, Ezer U, et al: Functional disability in children with hemophilic arthropathy, *Rheumatol Int* 26:1031, 2006.

H

41

❖

Hydrocephalus

Epidemiology

Hydrocephalus is a result of increased cerebrospinal fluid in the ventricles of the brain. Individuals with hydrocephalus are not able to absorb the excess cerebrospinal fluid. The excess fluid causes the ventricular spaces to widen and puts pressure on the cortex. Hydrocephalus can be classified as communicating or obstructive, depending on whether the cerebrospinal fluid is able to move between the ventricular spaces or not.

Nearly one in every 500 children will be born with or later acquire hydrocephalus. Acquired hydrocephalus is usually a secondary condition that results from an injury or insult to the brain.

Impact on Performance Skills

Children with hydrocephalus may experience difficulty in various motor, process, and communication and interaction skills depending on the areas of the brain that are affected and the reason for the hydrocephalus. Once a shunt is put in place, some of the performance deficits may subside.

Performance skills affected may include the following:
- Posture
- Mobility
- Coordination
- Strength and effort
- Energy

H

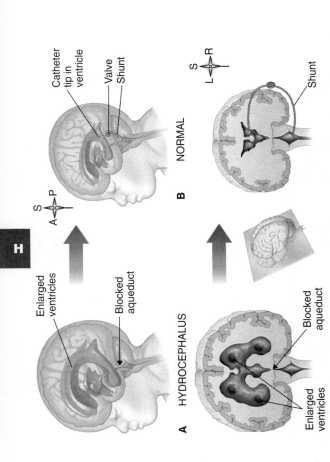

Hydrocephalus. **A,** Narrowing or blockage of the pathways for cerebrospinal fluid. **B,** This condition can be treated by the placement of a shunt to drain the excess fluid. (From Thibodeau GA, Patton KT: *The human body in health and disease,* ed 4, St Louis, 2005, Mosby.)

- Knowledge
- Temporal organization
- Organization of space and objects
- Adaptation
- Physicality
- Information exchange
- Relations

Performance patterns, such as habits, roles, and routines, may also be affected by hydrocephalus.

Impact on Client Factors (Body Functions and Structures)

Hydrocephalus may result in changes to the following client factors:

- Mental functions
- Sensory functions
- Movement-related functions

Precautions

Hydrocephalus may be seen secondary to a neurologic condition. Children who are at risk for hydrocephalus due to an insult or injury to the brain should be monitored for nausea, vomiting, seizures, complaints of blurred vision, motor incoordination, loss of balance, and change in energy levels.

Children who are receiving medical treatment for hydrocephalus often undergo intraventricular shunt placement. Intraventricular shunts help to relocate the built-up cerebrospinal fluid to another place in the body, where it can be more easily absorbed.

Children with intraventricular shunts should be monitored for shunt malfunction. Children who are experiencing shunt malfunction may demonstrate many of the signs and symptoms that are listed above.

Evaluation

- Clinical observations, including monitoring of signs and symptoms

- Interviews with child and family
- Assessment tools

Suggested Assessment Tools

- Alberta Infant Motor Scale (AIMS)
- Bayley Scale of Infant Development (BSID)
- Canadian Occupational Performance Measure (COPM)
- Children's Assessment of Participation and Enjoyment (CAPE)
- Denver Developmental Screening Test (DDST)
- Hawaii Early Learning Profile (HELP)
- Miller Function and Participation Scales (M-FUN-S)
- Peabody Developmental Motor Scales 2, Revised (PDMS-2)
- Pediatric Evaluation of Disability Inventory (PEDI)
- School Function Assessment (SFA)
- School Setting Interview (SSI)
- Short Child Occupational Profile (SCOPE)
- Toddler and Infant Motor Evaluation (TIME)
- WeeFIM

INTERVENTIONS

- Intervention to support the development of coordination, strength, and effort
- Support for participation in self-care and play
- Environmental accommodations and modifications
- Task accommodations and modifications
- Caregiver and family coaching
- Collaboration with other professionals

Case Example

The occupational therapist is working with Mr. Joseph and his 3-month-old infant, who recently underwent a surgical intraventricular shunt placement to treat hydrocephalus. Mr. Joseph is afraid to put his child on the floor to play because he is worried about shunt malfunction. The occupational therapist coaches Mr. Joseph on how to provide safe play opportunities for his child and educates him about signs to monitor for shunt malfunction. ❖

WEB RESOURCE

The National Institute of Neurological Disorders and Stroke
www.ninds.nih.gov/disorders/hydrocephalus/detail_hydrocephalus.htm

FURTHER READING

Fried A, Epstein M: Childhood hydrocephalus: clinical features, treatment, and the slit-ventricle syndrome. Available at: *www.virtualtrials.com/ shunts.cfm*. Accessed November 25, 2007.

H

42

❖

Hyperbilirubinemia

Epidemiology

Hyperbilirubinemia, or jaundice, is a condition in which there is too much bilirubin in the infant's blood. Approximately 60% of full-term infants and 80% of premature infants develop jaundice. Depending on the cause of the hyperbilirubinemia, jaundice may appear at birth or at any time afterward. Hyperbilirubinemia may be caused by numerous factors, including the following:

- Physiologic jaundice: as a response to an infant's typical ability to excrete bilirubin during the first days of life
- Breast milk jaundice: as a response to low calorie intake or dehydration
- Jaundice from hemolysis: as a response to Rh disease, having too many red blood cells, or bleeding
- Jaundice related to poor liver functioning: a result of liver malfunction or infection

Symptoms of hyperbilirubinemia or jaundice include the following:

- Yellow color of the infant's skin, usually beginning in the face
- Poor feeding
- Lethargy

Medical intervention for hyperbilirubinemia may include phototherapy—exposing the infant to special blue-spectrum

H

lights or covering the infant with a special fiberoptic blanket. Less conservative medical interventions include blood transfusions.

Impact on Client Factors (Body Functions and Structures)

- Hematologic functions

Precautions

If hyperbilirubinemia is not treated, large amounts of bilirubin may damage tissues in the brain and cause seizures or brain damage.

Infants who are undergoing phototherapy must have their eyes protected from the blue-spectrum lights. In addition, their body temperature should be monitored.

Evaluation

- Clinical observations
- Interview with family

INTERVENTION

- If infants with hyperbilirubinemia are receiving occupational therapy, it is likely because of another medical condition.

WEB RESOURCE
American Family Physician
www.aafp.org/afp/20020215/599.html

FURTHER READING
Weisiger R: Conjugated hyperbilirubinemia, 2007. Available at: *www. emedicine.com/med/topic1065.htm*. Accessed May 21, 2007.

43

❖

Hypoxic-Ischemic Encephalopathy

Epidemiology

Hypoxic-ischemic encephalopathy (HIE) is caused by brain injury due to asphyxia. The specific underlying causes of HIE are unknown. HIE may result in brain damage or even death. The duration and severity of the asphyxia is helpful in predicting long-term outcomes related to neurologic damage. It is estimated that two to four infants out of every 1000 will experience HIE. The mortality rate related to HIE is 50% to 75%.

Infants who survive HIE may have acquired brain injury, intellectual disabilities, epilepsy, or cerebral palsy.

Signs of HIE include the following:

- Hypotonia
- Poor feeding
- Irritability
- Disturbed sleep patterns
- Apnea
- Coma
- Absent neonatal reflexes
- Oculomotor disturbances
- Seizures
- Irregular heart rates
- Organ failure
- Pulmonary hypertension

Impact on Performance Skills

See chapters on Acquired Brain Injury, Intellectual Disabilities, Epilepsy, and Cerebral Palsy.

Impact on Client Factors (Body Functions and Structures)

See chapters on Acquired Brain Injury, Intellectual Disabilities, Epilepsy, and Cerebral Palsy.

Precautions

Most infants with HIE will require ventilator support during the first week of life. Blood pressure in infants with HIE should be monitored.

Evaluation

- Clinical observations
- Interviews with family and medical staff
- Assessment tools

Suggested Assessment Tools

See chapters on Acquired Brain Injury, Intellectual Disabilities, Epilepsy, and Cerebral Palsy.

INTERVENTION

- Infants and children might receive occupational therapy due to a condition caused by HIE. Please refer to entries for Acquired Brain Injury, Intellectual Disabilities, Epilepsy, or Cerebral Palsy.

WEB RESOURCE

Brain Injury Association of America
www.biausa.org

FURTHER READING

Chalak L, Kaiser J: Neonatal guideline hypoxic-ischemic encephalopathy (HIE), *J Ark Med Soc* 104:87, 2007.

Shah PS, Ohlsson A, Perlman M: Hypothermia to treat neonatal hypoxic ischemic encephalopathy: systematic review, *Arch Pediatr Adolesc Med* 161:951, 2007.

Gunn AJ, Gluckman PD: Head cooling for neonatal encephalopathy: the state of the art, *Clin Obstet Gynecol* 50:636, 2007.

H

44

Intellectual Disabilities

Epidemiology

Intellectual disabilities (IDs) are diagnosed based on a combination of three criteria:

- Intellectual functioning or IQ score below 70
- Significant limitations in adaptive skills
- Onset of the condition before age 18

ID has been linked to many causes, such as genetic disorders, metabolic disorders, prenatal complications, complications at birth, and severe early infancy fevers or infections. However, the three most common causes include Down syndrome, fragile X syndrome, and fetal alcohol syndrome.

Impact on Performance Skills

- Process skills
  - Energy
  - Knowledge
  - Temporal organization
  - Organization of space and objects
  - Adaptation
- Motor skills
  - Coordination
- Communication and interaction skills
  - Physicality
  - Information exchange
  - Relations

Impact on Client Factors (Body Functions and Structures)

- Global mental functions
- Specific mental functions

Precautions

No precautions have been noted.

Evaluation

- Clinical observations
- Interviews with child and family
- Assessment tools

Suggested Assessment Tools

- Alberta Infant Motor Scale (AIMS)
- Assessment of Motor and Process Skills (AMPS)
- Bayley Scale of Infant Development (BSID)
- Beery-Butenica Developmental Test of Visual Motor Integration (VMI)
- Benton Constructional Praxis Test
- Canadian Occupational Performance Measure (COPM)
- Child Occupational Self Assessment (COSA)
- Children's Assessment of Participation and Enjoyment (CAPE)
- Children's Handwriting Evaluation Scale (CHES)
- Denver Developmental Screening Test (DDST)
- Evaluation Tool of Children's Handwriting (ETCH)
- Gross Motor Function Measure (GMFM)
- Hawaii Early Learning Profile (HELP)
- Lincoln-Oseretsky Motor Development Scale
- Miller Function and Participation Scales (M-FUN-S)
- Movement Assessment Battery for Children (Movement ABC)
- Peabody Developmental Motor Scales 2 (PDMS-2)
- Pediatric Activity Card Sort (PACS)
- Pediatric Evaluation of Disability Inventory (PEDI)

- Pediatric Volitional Questionnaire (PVQ)
- Perceived Efficacy and Goal Setting System (PEGS)
- School Function Assessment (SFA)
- School Setting Interview (SSI)
- Sensory Processing Measure (SPM)
- Sensory Profile
- Short Child Occupational Profile (SCOPE)
- Toddler and Infant Motor Evaluation (TIME)
- Vineland Adaptive Behavior Scale
- WeeFIM

INTERVENTIONS

- Activities of daily living
- Instrumental activities of daily living
- Education
- Leisure
- Prevocational skills training
- Accommodations and modifications
- Support for the development of process skills
- Support for the development of motor and communication and interaction skills
- Environment and task accommodations and modifications
- Family coaching and training
- Support for the development of self-determination skills

Case Example

Jose is an 18-year-old with ID who resides in a group home. The occupational therapist works with Jose to teach him meal preparation skills. ❖

WEB RESOURCES

The Arc (a national organization on mental retardation)
www.thearc.org

American Association on Intellectual and Developmental Disabilities
www.aamr.org

FURTHER READING

Crowe TK, Florez SI: Time use of mothers with school-age children: a continuing impact of a child's disability, *Am J Occup Ther* 60:194, 2006.

45

❖

Intraventricular Hemorrhage

Epidemiology

Intraventricular hemorrhage (IVH) is bleeding inside or around the ventricles, the spaces in the brain containing the cerebral spinal fluid. IVH is most commonly seen in premature infants, especially those with low birth weight. IVH typically occurs within the first 3 days of life and is usually caused by complications related to prematurity. IVH causes permanent damage to nerve cells in the brain.

Bleeds related to IVH are graded based on their severity as follows:

- Grade I: bleeding occurs in just a small area of the ventricles
- Grade II: bleeding also occurs inside the ventricles
- Grade III: ventricles are enlarged by the blood
- Grade IV: bleeding into the brain tissues around the ventricles

Symptoms of IVH include the following:

- Disturbances in breathing, such as apnea and bradycardia
- Blue coloring or cyanosis
- Weak suck or difficulty feeding
- High-pitched cry
- Seizures
- Swelling or bulging of the fontanelles
- Low blood count or anemia

IVH may lead to intellectual disabilities, epilepsy, or cerebral palsy.

Impact on Performance Skills

See chapters on Intellectual Disabilities, Epilepsy, and Cerebral Palsy.

Impact on Client Factors (Body Functions and Structures)

See chapters on Intellectual Disabilities, Epilepsy, and Cerebral Palsy.

Precautions

See chapters on Intellectual Disabilities, Epilepsy, and Cerebral Palsy.

Evaluation

- Clinical observations
- Interviews with child and family
- Assessment tools

Suggested Assessment Tools

See chapters on Intellectual Disabilities, Epilepsy, and Cerebral Palsy.

INTERVENTION

- See chapters on Intellectual Disabilities, Epilepsy, and Cerebral Palsy.

Case Example

See chapters on Intellectual Disabilities, Epilepsy, and Cerebral Palsy. ❖

WEB RESOURCES

UCSF Children's Medical Hospital
www.ucsfhealth.org/childrens/health_professionals/manuals/49_IntraventricularHem.pdf

University of Michigan Health System
www.med.umich.edu/1libr/pa/pa_ivh_hhg.htm

FURTHER READING

Tortorolo G, Luciano R, Papacci P, Tonelli T: Intraventricular hemorrhage: past, present, and future, focusing on classification, pathogenesis, and prevention, *Child's Nerv Syst* 15:652, 1999.

I

46

❖

Juvenile Diabetes

Epidemiology

Diabetes is a medical condition in which the body has trouble regulating its blood glucose, or blood sugar, levels. There are two major types of diabetes, type 1 and type 2. Juvenile diabetes is considered type 1, or insulin-dependent, diabetes.

Type 1 diabetes causes the body's immune system to attack and destroy beta cells in the pancreas. In individuals without diabetes, beta cells produce insulin, a hormone that helps the body turn glucose into energy. However, when beta cells are destroyed, the pancreas cannot produce insulin and glucose stays in the blood instead. This can cause damage to the organ systems.

Medical intervention for individuals with type I diabetes includes taking insulin on a daily basis, either by injection or orally. In addition, individuals with diabetes must check their blood sugar levels several times per day and follow a carefully balanced diet. Individuals have to be careful to regulate their blood levels; otherwise they may develop hypoglycemia or hyperglycemia, which can be life-threatening.

Signs and symptoms of type 1 diabetes include the following:

- Extreme thirst
- Frequent urination
- Drowsiness or lethargy
- Sudden vision changes

- Changes in appetite
- Sudden weight loss
- Heavy, labored breathing
- States of unconsciousness

Type 1 diabetes is usually diagnosed in children, teenagers, or young adults.

Impact on Performance Patterns

Individuals with type 1 diabetes may need assistance to develop habits related to medical management of their condition.

Impact on Client Factors (Body Functions and Structures)

- Immunologic functions
- Hematologic functions

Precautions

Blood glucose levels must be measured regularly throughout the day; otherwise, individuals may develop hypoglycemia or hyperglycemia, which can be life-threatening.

Individuals with controlled type 1 diabetes will likely not require occupational therapy for this condition alone.

WEB RESOURCES

Juvenile Diabetes Research Foundation International
www.jdrf.org

Juvenile Diabetes Resource for Parents and Children
www.mychildhasdiabetes.com

FURTHER READING

Edmunds S, Roche D, Stratton G, et al: Physical activity and psychologic well-being in children with type 1 diabetes, *Psychol Health Med* 12:353, 2007.

47

Juvenile Rheumatoid Arthritis

Epidemiology

Juvenile rheumatoid arthritis (JRA) is the most common form of arthritis found in children and can vary in its level of severity. JRA affects girls twice as often as boys and can manifest anytime between birth and age 16.

The most common signs and symptoms of JRA include the following:

- Joint inflammation
- Joint contracture
- Joint damage
- Alteration in growth
- Stiffness
- Weakness in muscles around the affected joints

There are three major types of JRA:

- Pauciarticular, which affects four or fewer joints
- Polyarticular, which affects five or more joints
- Systemic, which affects at least one joint but causes inflammation of internal organs

Impact on Performance Skills

- Motor skills
  - Mobility
  - Coordination
  - Strength and effort

J

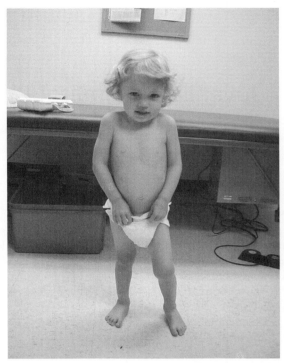

Pauciarticular juvenile rheumatoid arthritis. A 2-year-old girl with arthritis of the left knee. (From Zitelli BJ, Davis HW: *Atlas of pediatric physical diagnosis,* ed 5, St Louis, 2007, Mosby.)

J

Impact on Client Factors (Body Functions and Structures)

• Neuromusculoskeletal functions

Precautions

Children with JRA should not play contact sports or other sports that require repetitive motion. Children with JRA should also wear protective equipment whenever possible to reduce risk of injury.

Evaluation

- Clinical observations
- Interviews with child and family
- Assessment tools

Suggested Assessment Tools

- Assessment of Motor and Process Skills (AMPS)
- Canadian Occupational Performance Measure (COPM)
- Child Occupational Self Assessment (COSA)
- Miller Function and Participation Scales (M-FUN-S)
- Pediatric Activity Card Sort (PACS)
- Pediatric Evaluation of Disability Inventory (PEDI)
- Pediatric Interest Profile (PIP)
- Pediatric Volitional Questionnaire (PVQ)
- Perceived Efficacy and Goal Setting System (PEGS)
- School Function Assessment (SFA)
- School Setting Interview (SSI)
- Short Child Occupational Profile (SCOPE)
- WeeFIM

INTERVENTIONS

- Education on joint protection
- Accommodations and modifications for the task and the environment
- Range-of-motion exercises
- Strengthening for muscles around affected joints

J

Case Example

Judy is a 12-year-old student who is newly diagnosed with JRA. Judy's school-based occupational therapist makes recommendations to Judy and her teachers including the following:

- *Using built-up writing utensils*
- *Typing assignments and notes*
- *Recording lessons or photocopying another student's notes*

- *Shortening or modifying lengthy written assignments*
- *Using an adapted lock for her locker*
- *Preopening small packages of condiments in the cafeteria* ❖

WEB RESOURCES

Arthritis Foundation
www.arthritis.org

American College of Rheumatology
www.rheumatology.org

FURTHER READING

Nabors L, Iobst E, Weisnman J, et al: School support and functioning for children with juvenile rheumatic diseases, *J Dev Phys Disabil* 19:81, 2007.

48

❖

Klinefelter's Syndrome

Epidemiology

Klinefelter's syndrome is a medical condition of males who have an extra X chromosome. Klinefelter's syndrome affects approximately one of every 500 to 1000 newborn boys. Boys with Klinefelter's syndrome produce less than the typical amount of testosterone and may have less facial and body hair than other boys the same age.

Impact on Performance Skills

Individuals with Klinefelter's syndrome will likely not have difficulty with performance skills unless it is related to another medical condition.

Impact on Client Factors (Body Functions and Structures)

- Endocrine system functions

Precautions

No specific precautions are noted for Klinefelter's syndrome.

Evaluation

- Clinical observations
- Interviews with child and family
- Assessment tools

K

Suggested Assessment Tools

Individuals will not likely be receiving occupational therapy as a direct result of Klinefelter's syndrome. Occupational therapy practitioners should individualize the assessment plan for boys with Klinefelter's syndrome based on their unique presentation.

INTERVENTION

- Occupational therapy intervention will likely focus on addressing needs that are a result of a medical condition other than Klinefelter's syndrome. However, it is possible that some boys with Klinefelter's syndrome may experience self-esteem issues that are a result of their condition.

Case Example

Ryan is a 14-year-old boy with Klinefelter's syndrome. In the second quarter of the school year Ryan is brought to his school's prereferral team to address increased detentions as a result of fighting in the gym locker room. Ryan tells the social worker that the other boys have been teasing him, but he is unwilling to say more. During the prereferral team meeting, the school nurse indicates that Ryan has Klinefelter's syndrome. The occupational therapist suggests that Ryan be allowed to change in a private location rather than the crowded locker room. ❖

WEB RESOURCES

National Institute of Child Health and Human Development
www.nichd.nih.gov/publications/pubs/klinefelter.cfm

American Association for Klinefelter Syndrome and Support
www.aaksis.org

FURTHER READING

Sorensen K: Physical and mental development of adolescent males with Klinefelter syndrome, *Hormone Res* 37:55, 1992.

49

❖

Learning Disabilities

Epidemiology

Learning disabilities is an umbrella term used to refer to several neurologic disorders related to the way individuals learn. Individuals with learning disabilities have average or above-average intelligence but have difficulty with at least one of the following: reading, writing, language, spelling, math, reasoning, or processing.

It is estimated that approximately 15% of the population in the United States has a learning disability; difficulty with reading and language is the most common.

Some common learning disabilities include the following:

- Dyslexia: a language disability that usually manifests in difficulty with reading
- Dyscalculia: a math disability that usually manifests in difficulty computing problems or understanding math-related concepts
- Dysgraphia: a writing disability that manifests in difficulty with handwriting
- Auditory processing disorders: sensory-related disabilities that manifest in difficulty understanding language despite normal hearing
- Visual processing disorders: sensory-related disabilities that manifest in difficulty understanding written language and written math despite normal vision

L

Symptoms of learning disabilities vary with the expectations required of students with age. Some common signs and symptoms include the following:

- Delays in reaching developmental milestones, including those related to walking, talking, and self-care that has a large fine-motor component
- Difficulty learning numbers, letters, or shapes
- Difficulty with writing, drawing shapes, cutting, or coloring
- Difficulty following multistep directions or remembering information
- Difficulty learning letter sounds
- Spelling errors and letter or number reversals
- Delayed coordination or difficulty with motor planning
- Avoidance of homework; acting out in class

Impact on Performance Skills

- Process skills
  - Energy
    - Endures
    - Paces
    - Attends
  - Knowledge
    - Chooses
    - Uses
    - Handles
    - Heeds
    - Inquires
  - Temporal organization
    - Initiates
    - Continues
    - Sequences
    - Terminates
  - Organization of spaces and objects
    - Searches and locates
    - Gathers
    - Organizes

- Restores
- Navigates
- Adaptation
  - Notices and responds
  - Accommodates
  - Adjusts
  - Benefits
- Communication and interaction skills
  - Information exchange
    - Articulates
    - Asserts
    - Expresses
    - Speaks
    - Sustains
  - Relations
    - Collaborates
    - Conforms
    - Focuses

Impact on Client Factors (Body Functions and Structures)

- Specific mental functions
  - Attention functions
  - Memory functions
  - Perceptual functions
  - Higher-level cognitive functions
  - Mental functions of language
  - Calculation functions
  - Mental functions of sequencing complex movement
  - Experience of time functions

L

Precautions

When working with children with learning disabilities, it is easy to assume that their avoidance of certain tasks is related to noncompliant behavior. However, occupational therapy practitioners should determine whether the behavior truly is noncompliant or whether it signals difficulty with the task.

Evaluation

- Clinical observations
- Interviews with child and family
- Assessment tools

Suggested Assessment Tools

- Assessment of Communication and Interaction Skills (ACIS)
- Assessment of Motor and Process Skills (AMPS)
- Beery-Butenica Developmental Test of Visual-motor Integration (VMI)
- Behavioral Assessment of the Dysexecutive Syndrome (BADS)
- Canadian Occupational Performance Measure (COPM)
- Children's Handwriting Evaluation Scale (CHES)
- Children's Handwriting Evaluation Scale for Manuscript Writing (CHES-M)
- Coping Inventory
- Developmental Test of Visual Perception, Second Edition (DTVP-2)
- Digit Span
- Erhardt Developmental Prehension Assessment (EDPA)
- Erhardt Developmental Vision Assessment (EDVA)
- Evaluation Tool of Children's Handwriting (ETCH)
- Fine Motor Task Assessment
- Lowenstein Occupational Therapy Cognitive Assessment (LOTCA)
- Miller Assessment for Preschoolers (MAP)
- Miller Function and Participation Scales (M-FUN-S)
- Motor-free Visual Perceptual Test—Revised (MVPT-R)
- Pediatric Volitional Questionnaire (PVQ)
- School Assessment of Motor and Process Skills (School AMPS)
- School Function Assessment (SFA)
- School Setting Interview (SSI)
- Short Child Occupational Profile (SCOPE)
- Test of Everyday Attention for Children (TEA-Ch)
- Test of Handwriting Skills (THS)

- Test of Visual-Perceptual Skills (TVPS)
- Test of Visual-Motor Skills (TVMS)

INTERVENTIONS

- Support for formal educational participation
- Support for informal personal educational needs or interests
- Support for informal personal education
- Support for the development of process skills
- Support for the development of communication and interaction skills
- Environmental and task accommodations and modification
- Support for the development of perceptual skills
- Support for the development of skills related to academic tasks
- Teacher, parent, and child education

Case Example

Cal is a fourth-grade student who has been diagnosed with dyscalculia and dysgraphia. Cal struggles with math and has considerable difficulty lining up math problems and organizing the problems on his paper. The occupational therapist recommends that Cal copy down problems on graph paper and teaches him other strategies for organizing his paper. She also suggests that Cal be allowed to continue using manipulatives. ✢

WEB RESOURCES

LD Online
www.ldonline.org

Learning Disabilities Association of America
www.ldaamerica.org

FURTHER READING

Segal R, Hinojosa J: The activity setting of homework: an analysis of three cases and implications for occupational therapy, *Am J Occup Ther* 60:50, 2006.

L

50

Legg-Calvé-Perthes Disease

Epidemiology

Legg-Calvé-Perthes disease is a medical condition that is characterized by temporary loss of blood to the femoral head. It is also known as *ischemic necrosis of the hip*. This condition can occur anytime during childhood and is most common in boys 8 years old and younger.

Signs and symptoms of Legg-Calvé-Perthes disease include limping, leg length discrepancy, and pain and stiffness in the hip, groin, or knee. Children with Legg-Calvé-Perthes may develop osteoarthritis in adulthood.

Medical interventions for Legg-Calvé-Perthes disease include antiinflammatory drugs, surgery, bracing, and use of crutches or walking braces for ambulation.

Impact on Performance Skills

- Motor skills
  - Mobility
- Energy
  - Endures

Impact on Client Factors (Body Functions and Structures)

- Neuromusculoskeletal and movement-related functions

L

Precautions
No precautions have been noted.

Evaluation
- Clinical observations
- Interviews with child and family
- Assessment tools

Suggested Assessment Tools
- Children's Assessment of Participation and Enjoyment (CAPE)
- Denver Developmental Screening Test (DDST)
- Movement Assessment Battery for Children (Movement ABC)
- Peabody Developmental Motor Scale 2, Revised (PDMS-2)
- Pediatric Evaluation of Disability Inventory (PEDI)
- School Function Assessment (SFA)
- Short Child Occupational Profile (SCOPE)
- Test of Gross Motor Development (TGMD)
- WeeFIM

INTERVENTIONS
- Support for participation in activities of daily living
- Support for participation in play
- Environmental and task accommodations and modifications

L

Case Example
Ricky is a 4-year-old boy who was recently diagnosed with Legg-Calvé-Perthes disease. Ricky takes antiinflammatory medication and uses braces for walking. The occupational therapist provides her intervention at the playground and shows Ricky how he can play on the equipment safely while still using his braces. ❖

WEB RESOURCES

NIH/National Arthritis and Musculoskeletal and Skin Diseases
Information Clearinghouse
www.niams.nih.gov

March of Dimes
www.marchofdimes.com

FURTHER READING

Dutoit M: [Legg-Calvé-Perthes disease], *Arch Pediatr* 14:109, 2007.

L

51

❖

Lesch-Nyhan Syndrome

Epidemiology

Lesch-Nyhan syndrome is a rare genetic condition that is present at birth in baby boys and is caused by a deficiency of the enzyme hypoxanthine-guanine phosphoribosyltransferase (HPRT). The lack of HPRT causes a buildup of uric acid in all body fluids and leads to signs and symptoms such as severe gout, poor muscle control, and moderate intellectual disability, which appear in the first year of life.

Boys with Lesch-Nyhan syndrome may engage in self-harming behaviors, such as extreme lip, tongue, and finger biting. Other characteristics include facial grimacing, involuntary writhing, and repetitive movements of the arms and legs.

Impact on Performance Skills
- Motor skills
  - Posture
  - Mobility
  - Coordination
  - Strength and effort
  - Energy
- Process skills
  - Energy
  - Knowledge
  - Temporal organization

L

- Organization of space and objects
- Adaptation

Impact on Client Factors (Body Functions and Structures)

- Global mental functions
- Specific mental functions
- Muscle functions
- Movement functions

Precautions

Self-harming behaviors can lead to damage to anatomic structures and make structures more prone to infection.

Evaluation

- Clinical observations
- Interviews with child and family
- Assessment tools

Suggested Assessment Tools

- Alberta Infant Motor Scales (AIMS)
- Assessment of Motor and Process Skills (AMPS)
- Bayley Scale of Infant Development (BSID)
- Beery-Butenica Developmental Test of Visual Motor Integration (VMI)
- Benton Constructional Praxis Test
- Canadian Occupational Performance Measure (COPM)
- Child Occupational Self Assessment (COSA)
- Children's Assessment of Participation and Enjoyment (CAPE)
- Children's Handwriting Evaluation Scale (CHES)
- Denver Developmental Screening Test (DDST)
- Evaluation Tool of Children's Handwriting (ETCH)
- Gross Motor Function Measure (GMFM)
- Hawaii Early Learning Profile (HELP)
- Lincoln-Oseretsky Motor Development Scale
- Miller Function and Participation Scales (M-FUN-S)

- Movement Assessment Battery for Children (Movement ABC)
- Peabody Developmental Motor Scales 2, Revised (PDMS-2)
- Pediatric Activity Card Sort (PACS)
- Pediatric Evaluation of Disability Inventory (PEDI)
- Perceived Efficacy and Goal Setting System (PEGS)
- School Function Assessment (SFA)
- School Setting Interview (SSI)
- Short Child Occupational Profile (SCOPE)
- Toddler and Infant Motor Evaluation (TIME)
- Vineland Adaptive Behavior Scale (VABS)
- WeeFIM

INTERVENTIONS

- Activities of daily living
- Instrumental activities of daily living
- Education
- Leisure
- Prevocational skills training
- Accommodations and modifications
- Support for the development of muscle strength and motor coordination
- Support for the development of process skills
- Environment and task accommodations and modifications
- Family coaching and training
- Support for the development of self-determination skills

L

Case Example

Vernell is a 3-year-old boy with Lesch-Nyhan syndrome who attends a half-day early childhood program. The occupational therapist works with Vernell on increasing fine motor strength and coordination so that he can complete art projects and play at various centers with his peers. ❖

WEB RESOURCE

National Institute of Neurological Disorders and Stroke
www.ninds.nih.gov/disorders/lesch_nyhan/lesch_nyhan.htm

FURTHER READING

Jimenez R, Puig J: Rare diseases: Lesch-Nyhan syndrome, *Med Clin (Barc)* 122:358, 2004.

L

52

Lordosis

Epidemiology

Lordosis is a condition characterized by an excessive inward curve of the spine, usually seen in the lumbar region. Lordosis may be caused by other conditions such as kyphosis, achondroplasia, obesity, or spondylolisthesis.

Medical interventions for lordosis include both surgical and nonsurgical treatment.

Surgical intervention is considered only when the lordotic curve is so severe that it affects the spinal nerves or when nonsurgical intervention has not worked. Nonsurgical intervention includes analgesics, antiinflammatory medication, physical therapy to build strength and increase flexibility, bracing to prevent further progression, and diet and exercise to reduce obesity.

Impact on Performance Skills

- Motor skills
  - Posture
  - Mobility
  - Coordination
  - Strength and effort

Impact on Client Factors (Body Functions and Structures)

- Neuromusculoskeletal functions

L

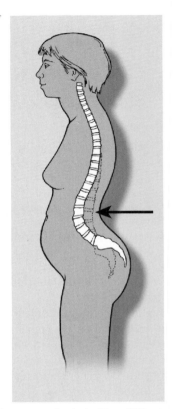

Abnormal spinal curvature: lordosis. (From Thibodeau GA, Patton KT: *The human body in health and disease,* ed 4, St Louis, 2005, Mosby.)

L

Precautions

Bracing and proper positioning might be required to prevent further development of the curve.

Evaluation

- Clinical observations
- Interviews with child and family
- Assessment tools

Suggested Assessment Tools

- Assessment of Motor and Process Skills (AMPS)
- Canadian Occupational Performance Measure (COPM)
- Child Occupational Self Assessment (COSA)
- Miller Function and Participation Scales (M-FUN-S)
- Pediatric Activity Card Sort (PACS)
- Pediatric Evaluation of Disability Inventory (PEDI)
- Pediatric Interest Profile (PIP)
- Pediatric Volitional Questionnaire (PVQ)
- Perceived Efficacy and Goal Setting System (PEGS)
- School Function Assessment (SFA)
- School Setting Interview (SSI)
- Short Child Occupational Profile (SCOPE)
- WeeFIM

INTERVENTIONS

- Support for activities of daily living
- Support for instrumental activities of daily living
- Task and environment accommodations and modifications
- Provision of training for use of adaptive equipment
- Recommendations for positioning

Case Example

June, a 15-year-old girl with achondroplasia, was recently admitted to the hospital to have corrective surgery for severe lordosis. After surgery June must wear a rigid thoracic-lumbar-sacral orthosis (TLSO) brace. Because she is unable to bend her back, the occupational therapist works with June to complete self-care activities of daily living and recommends adaptive equipment, such as a reacher. ❖

WEB RESOURCES

American Physical Therapy Association
www.apta.org

American Chiropractic Association
www.acatoday.com/content_css.cfm?CID=2189

FURTHER READING

Carter E, Davis J, Raggio C: Advances in understanding etiology of achondroplasia and review of management, *Curr Opin Pediatr* 19:32, 2007.

Lipton G, Letonoff E, Dabney K, et al: Correction of sagittal plane spinal deformities with unit rod instrumentation in children with cerebral palsy, *J Bone Joint Surg Am* 85:2349, 2003.

L

53

❖

Marfan Syndrome

Epidemiology

Marfan syndrome is an inheritable disorder of connective tissue, the tissue that strengthens the body's structures. Connective tissue disorders affect the skeletal system, cardio-vascular system, eyes, and skin.

Marfan syndrome is inherited as an autosomal dominant trait. Many cases are associated with no family history and are spontaneous new mutations. The mutation is in the gene that encodes fibrillin-1. Fibrillin-1 plays an important role as the scaffolding for elastic tissue in the body; in particular the changes occur in the aorta, eyes and skin. The mutations also cause overgrowth of the long bones of the body, resulting in the tall stature and long limbs seen in clients with Marfan syndrome.

Impact on Performance Skills

Children with Marfan syndrome may have motor skill delays in the following areas:

- Posture
- Coordination
- Strength and effort
- Energy

Typically, children with Marfan syndrome will not demonstrate delays in process or communication and interaction skills.

M

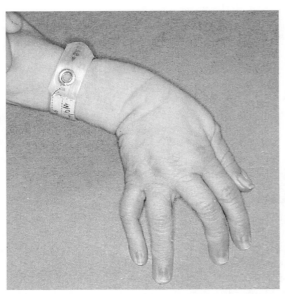

In Marfan syndrome, fingers, arms, legs, and toes may be dispropor-
tionately long in relation of the rest of the body, as in this infant.
(From Zitelli BJ, Davis HW: *Atlas of pediatric physical diagnosis,* ed 5,
St Louis, 2007, Mosby.)

Impact on Client Factors (Body Functions and Structures)

Children with Marfan syndrome are often tall and thin and
may have heart problems. They also may have slender, taper-
ing fingers, long arms and legs, curvature of the spine, and
eye problems. Sometimes the Marfan syndrome is so mild
that few (if any) symptoms occur. In the most severe cases,
which are rare, life-threatening problems may occur at
any age.

Marfan syndrome causes skeletal defects such as a tall,
lanky frame, long limbs and spider-like fingers, chest abnormalities, curvature of the spine, and a particular set of facial

features, including a highly arched palate and crowded teeth.

Common eye problems include nearsightedness and dislocation of the eye's lens.

Precautions
Impact on Performance Skills
Visual deficits could potentially interfere with performance of daily and school activities. Children with Marfan syndrome also may have heart problems that limit ability to participate in physical activities. This could affect ability to play or participate in extracurricular activities.

Impact on Client Factors (Body Functions and Structures)
The most significant of the defects in the syndrome are cardiovascular abnormalities, which may include enlargement of the base of the aorta, with aortic regurgitation, and prolapse of the mitral valve. This could cause fatigue and limit participation, causing poor heart function.

Evaluation
• Observations related to home, school, and community accessibility

Suggested Assessment Tools
• Canadian Occupational Performance Measure (COPM)
• Short Child Occupational Profile (SCOPE)

INTERVENTION
• Environmental accommodations and modifications

M

Case Example
Ethan is referred to occupational therapy because his mother said he has difficulty moving food around in his mouth and swallowing.

The occupational therapist identifies that this is most likely related to structural issues in Ethan's mouth and helps the mother to adapt feeding to meet Ethan's needs. ❖

WEB RESOURCE
National Marfan Foundation
www.marfan.orgnmf/index.jsp

FURTHER READING

Aburawi EH, O'Sullivan J, Hasan A: Marfan's syndrome: a review, *Hosp Med* 62:153, 2001.

Dean JC: Marfan syndrome: clinical diagnosis and management, *Eur J Hum Genet* 15:724, 2007.

'Ryan-Krause P: Identify and manage Marfan syndrome in children, *Nurse Pract* 27:26, 2002.

Strider D, Moore T, Guarini J, et al: Marfan's syndrome: a family affair, *J Vasc Nurs,* 14:91, 1996.

M

54

❖

Meconium Aspiration Syndrome

Epidemiology

Meconium is the first feces (stool) of the newborn. It is thick, sticky, and greenish black. A child can aspirate this mixture either in the uterus or just after delivery. During a stressful labor an infant may experience a lack of oxygen. This can cause increased movement of the infant's intestines and relaxation of the anal sphincter, causing meconium to pass into the amniotic fluid surrounding the unborn baby.

The inhaled meconium can partially or completely block the infant's airways. This may cause problems for the infant such as pneumonia or other breathing problems. It can also cause limitations in motor skills, sensory processing, and communication and interaction skills.

Impact on Performance Skills

Children with meconium aspiration may have delays in motor skills such as the following:

M

- Posture
- Mobility
- Coordination
- Strength and effort
- Energy

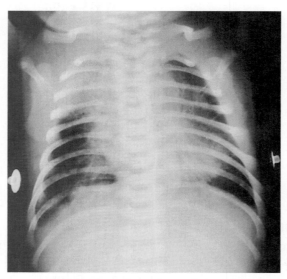

Meconium aspiration. The radiograph reveals irregularly distributed areas of hyperaeration and consolidation. (From Zitelli BJ, Davis HW: *Atlas of pediatric physical diagnosis,* ed 5, St Louis, 2007, Mosby.)

Typically children with meconium aspiration will not demonstrate delays in process or communication and interaction skills.

Impact on Client Factors
- Movement-related functions
- Sensory functions

Precautions

Impact on Performance Skills
Some children with meconium aspiration may experience a shortage of oxygen to the brain, which can affect the child's motor skills as well as sensory skills. It can also affect their interactions with their parents.

Impact on Client Factors (Body Functions and Structures)

Children with meconium aspiration are at risk for having sensory issues as well as impairment to neuromuscular functioning.

Evaluation

- Clinical observations
- Interviews with family and health care providers
- Assessment tools

Suggested Assessment Tools

- Bayley Scales of Infant Development (BSID)
- Denver Developmental Screening Test (DDST)
- Early Coping Inventory
- Erhardt Developmental Prehension Assessment (EDPA)
- Erhardt Developmental Vision Assessment, Revised (EDVA)
- Hawaii Early Learning Profile (HELP)
- Infant/Toddler Sensory Profile
- Knox Preschool Play Scale
- Movement Assessment for Infants (MAI)
- Peabody Developmental Motor Scales 2, Revised (PDMS-2)
- Short Child Occupational Profile (SCOPE)
- Toddler and Infant Motor Evaluation (TIME)
- Vineland Adaptive Behavior Scales, Revised (VABS)

INTERVENTIONS

- Environmental accommodations and modifications
- Task accommodations and modifications
- Intervention to increase mobility, posture, coordination, and strength
- Tone management
- Caregiver and family coaching

M

Case Example

Jaelyn, a 1-year-old girl, is being seen by an occupational therapist because of poor postural control as a result of meconium aspiration. The occupational therapist works with the toddler's parents to identify issues in the home environment and provides a program for them to use that will also complement the interventions that the occupational therapist provides during in-home visits. ❖

WEB RESOURCE

Kids Health for Parents
www.kidshealth.orgparent/medical/lungs/meconium.html

FURTHER READING

Dargaville PA, Copnell B, Australian and New Zealand Neonatal Network: The epidemiology of meconium aspiration syndrome: incidence, risk factors, therapies, and outcome, *Pediatrics* 117:1712, 2006.

Greenough A, Pulikot A, Dimitriou G: Prevention and management of meconium aspiration syndrome—assessment of evidence based practice, *Eur J Pediatr* 164:329, 2005.

Keenan WJ: Recommendations for management of the child born through meconium-stained amniotic fluid, *Pediatrics* 113:133, 2004.

Moore CS: Meconium aspiration syndrome, *Neonatal Netw* 19:41, 2000.

Srinivasan HB, Vidyasagar D: Meconium aspiration syndrome: current concepts and management, *Compr Ther* 25:82, 1999.

M

55

❖

Micrognathia

Epidemiology

Micrognathia is a small lower jaw. Micrognathia may be the only abnormality in a child. It is often self-correcting as a child grows. This is especially true at puberty, when the jaw grows significantly. This may also be seen in children with certain inherited disorders and syndromes.

Impact on Performance Skills

Children with micrognathia may have delays in motor skills (oral control), such as the following:
- Mobility
- Coordination
- Strength and effort

Also, children may experience delays in communication and interaction skills such as the following:
- Information exchange

Typically children with micrognathia will not demonstrate delays in process skills.

Impact on Client Factors (Body Functions and Structures)

Micrognathia can be enough to interfere with feeding because the jaw is so small. Feeding adaptations may be necessary.

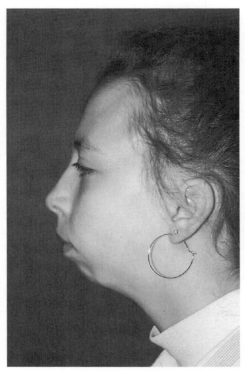

Micrognathia. Note the underdevelopment of the jaw and retracted chin. (From Zitelli BJ, Davis HW: *Atlas of pediatric physical diagnosis,* ed 5, St Louis, 2007, Mosby.)

Precautions

Impact on Performance Skills

A child with micrognathia can have issues that interfere with feeding. Techniques can be learned through special programs that focus on issues related to oral structural problems or sensory issues.

Impact on Client Factors (Body Functions and Structures)

Micrognathia is one cause of abnormal alignment of the teeth. The child or infant will have trouble with teeth closure. Many times there is not enough room for the teeth to grow, and a dental consultation is helpful.

Evaluation

- Clinical observations
- Observations related to feeding
- Interviews with the family
- Sensory processing

Suggested Assessment Tools

- Canadian Occupational Performance Measure (COPM)
- Child Occupational Self-Assessment (COSA)
- Infant/Toddler Sensory Profile
- Pediatric Evaluation of Disability Inventory (PEDI)
- Pediatric Volitional Questionnaire (PVQ)
- Short Child Occupational Profile (SCOPE)

INTERVENTIONS

- Special feeding techniques and equipment
- Feeding accommodations and modifications
- Oral desensitization

Case Example

Joseph, a toddler, is being seen in the occupational therapy clinic for issues related to trisomy 13. His mother is concerned because he is having trouble eating because of micrognathia. She has asked the occupational therapist if there is anything that can be done. The occupational therapist provides adaptations to feeding and explores any issues that may be due to sensory problems. ❖

M

WEB RESOURCE

Genetics Home Reference
**http://ghr.nlm.nih.gov/ghr/glossary/micrognathia;jsessionid=
61B91B1CA96E268163B72BA01B4B318B**

FURTHER READING

Elliott MA, Studen-Pavlovich DA, Ranalli DN: Prevalence of selected pediatric conditions in children with Pierre Robin sequence, *Pediatr Dent* 17:106, 1995.

van der Haven I, Mulder JW, van der Wal KG, et al: The jaw index: new guide defining micrognathia in newborns, *Cleft Palate Craniofac J* 34:240, 1997.

56

❖

Mononucleosis

Epidemiology

Mononucleosis is a viral infection causing fevers, sore throat, and swollen lymph glands, especially in the neck. It is usually linked to the Epstein-Barr virus (EBV) but can also be caused by other organisms such as cytomegalovirus (CMV).

Mononucleosis is often transmitted by saliva. Although it is known as "the kissing disease," occurring most often in 15- to 17-year-olds, the infection may occur at any age.

Mononucleosis can begin with fatigue, malaise, headache, and sore throat. The sore throat slowly gets worse, often with swollen tonsils. The lymph nodes in the neck are frequently swollen and painful. The symptoms of mononucleosis gradually go away over a period of weeks to months.

Impact on Performance Skills

Children with mononucleosis may have delays in motor skills such as the following:
- Strength and effort
- Energy

They may also experience delays in process skills such as the following:
- Energy

Typically children with mononucleosis will not demonstrate delays in communication and interaction skills.

M

Impact on Client Factors (Body Functions and Structures)

Because of the fatigue and general malaise related to mononucleosis, children have a difficult time maintaining the energy levels necessary to participate in or complete activities.

Precautions

Impact on Performance Skills

Some children have a difficult time participating in their normal daily activities and must be placed on restrictive activity and rest cycles. This can affect the strength and effort that a child generates during occupations.

Impact on Client Factors (Body Functions and Structures)

Children with mononucleosis can have problems maintaining energy during activities, which results in possible problems with muscle and movement functions.

Evaluation

- Checklists, observations, and formal assessments related to performance skills in the home, school, and community
- Interviews with the child and family

Suggested Assessment Tools

- Assessment of Motor and Process Skills (AMPS)
- Bay Area Functional Performance Evaluation (BaFPE)
- Bruininks-Oseretsky Test of Motor Proficiency
- Canadian Occupational Performance Measure (COPM)
- Child Occupational Self Assessment (COSA)
- NIH Activity Record
- Occupational Performance History Inventory (OPHI)
- Short Child Occupational Profile (SCOPE)

INTERVENTIONS

- Environmental accommodations and modifications
- Task accommodations and modifications
- Energy conservation education

Case Example

Patricia, a 15-year-old with mononucleosis, is a sophomore in high school. She is involved in multiple extracurricular activities as well as having responsibilities at home. She consulted with the school occupational therapist to determine methods for energy conservation. ❖

WEB RESOURCE

Mayo Clinic
www.mayoclinic.com/health/mononucleosis/DS00352

FURTHER READING

Belkengren R, Sapala S: Pediatric management problems. Infectious mono-
    nucleosis, *Pediatr Nurs* 28:259, 2002.

Charles PG: Infectious mononucleosis, *Aust Fam Physician* 32:785, 2003.

Papesch M, Watkins R: Epstein-Barr virus infectious mononucleosis, *Clin
    Otolaryngol Allied Sci* 26:3, 2001.

Peter J, Ray CG: Infectious mononucleosis, *Pediatr Rev* 19:276, 1998.

M

57

❖

Muscular Dystrophy

Epidemiology

Muscular dystrophy (MD) refers to a group of more than 30 inherited diseases that cause muscle weakness and muscle loss. Some forms of MD appear in infancy or childhood, whereas others may not appear until middle age or later. The different muscular dystrophies vary in symptoms and in whom they affect.

All forms of MD grow worse as the person's muscles get weaker. Most people with MD eventually lose the ability to walk. There is no cure for MD, but medications and therapy can slow the course of the disease.

The most common types of MD appear to be due to a genetic deficiency of the muscle protein dystrophin. Muscles, primarily voluntary muscles, become progressively weaker. In the late stages of MD, fat and connective tissue often replace muscle fibers. In some types of MD, heart muscles, other involuntary muscles, and other organs are affected.

Dystrophinopathies

Dystrophinopathies are due to a genetic deficiency of the protein dystrophin.

Duchenne Muscular Dystrophy

Duchenne MD is the most severe form of dystrophinopathy. It occurs mostly in young boys and is the most common form of MD that affects children.

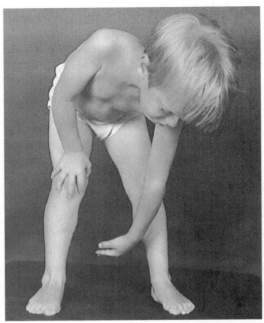

A boy with Duchenne muscular dystrophy. This child has difficulty rising from the floor. (From Zitelli BJ, Davis HW: *Atlas of pediatric physical diagnosis,* ed 5, St Louis, 2007, Mosby.)

Myotonic Dystrophy

Myotonic dystrophy is also known as *Steinert's disease.* This form of MD produces stiffness of muscles and an inability to relax muscles at will.

Facioscapulohumeral Muscular Dystrophy

Facioscapulohumeral MD is also known as *Landouzy-Dejerine disease.* This form involves progressive muscle weakness, usually in this order: face, shoulders, abdomen, feet, upper arms, pelvic area, and lower arms.

Impact on Performance Skills

Children with MD may have delays in motor skills such as the following:

- Posture
- Mobility
- Coordination
- Strength and effort
- Energy

Children with MD may experience delays in process skills such as the following:

- Energy
- Knowledge
- Temporal organization
- Adaptation

Children with MD may experience delays in communication and interaction skills such as the following:

- Physicality
- Information exchange

Impact on Client Factors (Body Functions and Structures)

In general MD results in frequent falls, apparent lack of coordination, muscle weakness, progressive crippling (resulting in contractures of the muscles around the joints), loss of mobility, difficulty getting up from a lying or sitting position, weakness in lower leg muscles (resulting in difficulty running and jumping), waddling gait, and mild intellectual disabilities (in some cases). This causes problems for a child by limiting participation in activities and tasks without adaptations to tasks or the environment.

The signs and symptoms of the multiple forms of MD differ. Each type is different in the age of onset, what parts of the body the symptoms primarily affect, and how rapidly the disease progresses.

M

Precautions

Impact on Performance Skills

MD can cause children to have problems with swallowing, coordination, muscle strength, and limb use, which can affect motor skills. Some forms of MD can cause mild intellectual disabilities, and this can affect functioning in certain contexts if not identified.

Impact on Client Factors (Body Functions and Structures)

Some children with Duchenne MD may exhibit curvature of the spine (scoliosis).

Evaluation

- Checklists or observations related to home, school, and community related to access and child-environment fit
- Interviews with the child, family, teachers, other professionals

Suggested Assessment Tools

- Assessment of Motor and Process Skills (AMPS)
- Balcones Sensory Integration Screening Kit
- Bay Area Functional Performance Evaluation (BaFPE)
- Box and Block Test
- Bruininks-Oseretsky Test of Motor Proficiency (BOT-2)
- Canadian Occupational Performance Measure (COPM)
- Children's Assessment of Participation and Enjoyment (CAPE)
- Choosing Outcomes and Accommodations for Children (COACH)
- Classroom Observation Guide
- Fine Motor Task Assessment
- Hawaii Early Learning Profile (HELP)
- Klein-Bell Activities of Daily Living Scale
- Lincoln-Oseretsky Motor Development Scale
- Pediatric Evaluation of Disability Inventory (PEDI)

M

- School Function Assessment (SFA)
- Short Child Occupational Profile (SCOPE)
- Toddler and Infant Motor Evaluation (TIME)
- Vineland Adaptive Behavior Scales Revised (VABS)
- WeeFIM

INTERVENTIONS

- Environmental accommodations and modifications
- Task accommodations and modifications
- Positioning in the home, school, and community in strollers, wheelchairs, and classroom chairs
- Interest exploration for leisure participation

Case Example

Johnny is an 8-year-old with Duchenne MD. His mother requested an occupational therapist to consult in the home to help determine modifications to the environment to accommodate Johnny's wheelchair. The OT has made a number of recommendations regarding width of doorways and the entry way into the home to accommodate Johnny's wheelchair. The family has limited resources, so the occupational therapist is working with a social worker to help the family find assistance to make the necessary modifications. ❖

WEB RESOURCE

Muscular Dystrophy Association
www.mdausa.org

FURTHER READING

Kakulas BA: Problems and solutions in the rehabilitation of patients with progressive muscular dystrophy, *Scand J Rehabil Med Suppl* 39:23, 1999.

Siegel IM: Muscular dystrophy: multidisciplinary approach to management, *Postgrad Med* 69:124, 1981.

Strober JB: Genetics of pediatric neuromuscular disease, *Curr Opin Pediatr* 12:549, 2000.

M

58

❖

Necrotizing Enterocolitis

Epidemiology

Necrotizing enterocolitis is an acquired disease in which intestinal tissue dies and the tissue sloughs off. It occurs primarily in premature infants or sick newborns. The cause for this disorder is unknown, but it is thought to be related to a decreased blood flow to the bowel. This keeps the bowel from producing the normal protective mucus. Bacteria in the intestine may also be a cause.

Necrotizing enterocolitis has a high death rate, but the outcome of the disease can be improved with early and aggressive treatment. Small, premature infants who are fed concentrated formulas, infants in a nursery where an outbreak has occurred (suggesting an infectious cause), or infants who have received blood exchange transfusions are at risk for necrotizing enterocolitis.

Impact on Performance Skills

Children with necrotizing enterocolitis may have delays in motor skills such as the following:

- Posture
- Mobility
- Strength and effort
- Energy

Children with necrotizing enterocolitis may experience delays in process skills such as the following:

N

- Energy
- Temporal organization
- Adaptation

Typically children with necrotizing enterocolitis will not demonstrate delays in communication and interaction skills.

Impact on Client Factors (Body Functions and Structures)

Infants suspected of having necrotizing enterocolitis will have feedings stopped and gas relieved from the bowel through insertion of a small tube into the stomach. Intravenous fluid replaces other forms of liquid such as formula or breast milk. Antibiotic therapy is started, and the infant's condition is monitored with abdominal x-ray examinations, blood tests, and assessment of blood gases. This can affect an infant's oral sensory processing.

Precautions

Impact on Performance Skills

Some infants have necrotizing enterocolitis that results in abdominal distention, vomiting and feeding intolerance, blood in the stool (visible or microscopic), lethargy, temperature instability, diarrhea, intestinal perforation, sepsis, peritonitis, and intestinal stricture (a narrow area that may lead to bowel obstruction). This can affect the infant's ability to have the motor skills necessary to participate in activities that are part of infancy.

Impact on Client Factors (Body Functions and Structures)

Infants may have surgery if there is an intestinal hole or inflammation of the abdominal wall. Surgery removes the dead bowel tissue, and a colostomy is performed. After the infection and inflammation have healed, the bowel is reconnected, which can take several weeks or months. This leaves the infant at risk for low weight, which leads to poor energy and ability and in the likelihood that there will be delays in developing motor, process, and interaction skills.

Evaluation
- Clinical observation
- Family and caregiver interviews
- Infant-environment fit and interaction

Suggested Assessment Tools
- Alberta Infant Motor Scales (AIMS)
- Denver Developmental Screening Test (DDST)
- Early Coping Inventory
- Infant/Toddler Sensory Profile
- Mother-Child Interaction Checklist
- Movement Assessment for Infants (MAI)
- Peabody Developmental Motor Scales 2, Revised (PDMS-2)
- Pediatric Evaluation of Disability Inventory (PEDI)
- Short Child Occupational Profile (SCOPE)
- Toddler and Infant Motor Evaluation (TIME)
- Vineland Adaptive Behavior Scales Revised (VABS)
- WeeFIM

INTERVENTIONS
- Task accommodations and modifications
- Sensory modulation
- Parental and caregiver training
- Feeding

Case Example

Josie, a toddler in day care, was exposed to and picked up necrotizing enterocolitis. She has lost a lot of weight, and the occupational therapist who is working with Josie has identified that Josie is experiencing delays in preacademic skills because of low levels of energy and decreased participation in motor activities. The occupational

N

therapist will provide therapy and a home program for the family to carry out to help improve Josie's motor delays. ❖

WEB RESOURCES

NCT Info Center
www.nct.org.uk/info/Necrotizing_Entercolitis

March of Dimes
www.marchofdimes.com/newsletters/February_2004.asp

FURTHER READING

Hall N, Pierro A: Necrotizing enterocolitis, *Hosp Med,* 65:220, 2004.

Horton KK: Pathophysiology and current management of necrotizing enterocolitis, *Neonatal Netw* 24:37, 2005.

Henry MC, Moss RL: Current issues in the management of necrotizing enterocolitis, *Semin Perinatol* 28:221, 2004.

Smith JR: Early enteral feeding for the very low birth weight infant: the development and impact of a research-based guideline, *Neonatal Netw* 24:9, 2005.

59

❖

Neonatal Respiratory Distress Syndrome

Epidemiology

Respiratory distress syndrome is one of the most common lung disorders in premature infants and rarely affects full-term infants. The condition makes it difficult to breathe.

The disease occurs when the lungs lack a chemical (lung surfactant) that helps them inflate with air and keeps the air sacs from collapsing. Lung surfactant appears in mature lungs. Respiratory distress syndrome usually appears shortly after birth and slowly becomes more severe.

Impact on Performance Skills

Infants who have experienced respiratory distress may have delays in motor skills such as the following:

- Posture
- Mobility
- Coordination
- Strength and effort
- Energy

Infants who have experienced respiratory distress may have delays in process skills such as the following:

- Energy
- Knowledge
- Temporal organization

N

- Organization of space and objects
- Adaptation

Infants who have experienced respiratory distress may have delays in communication and interaction skills such as the following:

- Physicality
- Information exchange

Impact on Client Factors (Body Functions and Structures)

Long-term complications may develop as a result of oxygen toxicity, high pressures delivered to the lungs, the severity of the condition itself, or periods when the brain or other organs did not receive enough oxygen. This can cause a child to have problems with motor skills, sensory processing, and participation in tasks as the infant grows and develops.

Precautions

Impact on Performance Skills

Some infants with respiratory distress experience pneumothorax, pneumomediastinum, pneumopericardium, or bronchopulmonary dysplasia, and this can affect motor, process, and communication and interaction skills, with both short- and long-term implications.

Impact on Client Factors (Body Functions and Structures)

Infants with respiratory distress are at risk for brain hemorrhage (intraventricular bleed), hemorrhage into the lung (sometimes associated with surfactant use), thrombotic events associated with an umbilical arterial catheter, retrolental fibroplasia and blindness, delayed mental development, and intellectual disabilities associated with anoxic brain damage or hemorrhage. This can lead to general and specific developmental delays.

Evaluation

- Clinical observations
- Interviews with family and care providers

Suggested Assessment Tools

- Alberta Infant Motor Scales (AIMS)
- Bayley Scales of Infant Development (BSID)
- Early Coping Inventory
- Erhardt Developmental Prehension Assessment (EDPA)
- Erhardt Developmental Vision Assessment Revised (EDVA)
- Gross Motor Function Measure (GMFM)
- Hawaii Early Learning Profile (HELP)
- Home Observation and Measurement of the Environment (HOME)
- Infant/Toddler Sensory Profile
- Knox Preschool Play Scale
- Movement Assessment for Infants (MAI)
- Peabody Developmental Motor Scales 2, Revised (PDMS-2)
- Pediatric Evaluation of Disability Inventory (PEDI)
- Short Child Occupational Profile (SCOPE)
- Toddler and Infant Motor Evaluation (TIME)
- Vineland Adaptive Behavior Scales Revised (VABS)

INTERVENTIONS

- Joint protection measures through positioning to reduce possible deformity and pain
- Sensory skills to decrease likelihood of sensory deprivation
- Family relational needs
- Enhancement of motor control and skills, both fine and gross motor
- Increase interest in and attention to play activities

N

Case Example

Mya is a newborn who experienced neonatal respiratory distress. She has been placed in an incubator with limited human contact. There is a concern that she will experience deformities in her extremities as a result of poor positioning. The occupational therapist has evaluated Mya and designed and implemented a positioning program for her to be carried out during her stay in the incubator. ❖

WEB RESOURCE

BIObank
http://lib.bioinfo.pl/meid:19337

FURTHER READING

Hermansen CL, Lorah KN: Respiratory distress in the newborn, *Am Fam Physician* 76:987, 2007.

Meade MO, Herridge MS: An evidence-based approach to acute respiratory distress syndrome, *Respir Care* 46:1368, 2001.

Wells DA, Gillies D, Fitzgerald DA: Positioning for acute respiratory distress in hospitalised infants and children, *Cochrane Database Syst Rev* Apr 18: CD003645, 2005.

N

60

❖

Neurofibromatosis

Epidemiology

Neurofibromatosis type 1, also called *von Recklinghausen's disease*, is a rare genetic disorder characterized by the development of multiple benign tumors of nerves and skin and areas of abnormally decreased or increased coloration of the skin. Areas of abnormal pigmentation typically include pale tan or light brown discolorations on the skin of the trunk and other regions as well as freckling, particularly under the arms and in the groin area.

Affected children manifest such conditions as early as 1 year of age, and the changes tend to increase in size and number over time. Neurofibromatosis takes two different forms: type 1 (NF-1) and type 2 (NF-2). One abnormal gene causes each form.

Impact on Performance Skills

Children with neurofibromatosis may experience delays in motor skills such as the following:

- Posture
- Mobility
- Coordination
- Strength and effort
- Energy

Children with neurofibromatosis may experience delays in process skills such as the following:

N

- Energy
- Temporal organization
- Organization of space and objects
- Adaptation

Children with neurofibromatosis may experience delays in communication and interaction skills such as the following:

- Physicality
- Information exchange
- Relations

Impact on Client Factors (Body Functions and Structures)

At birth or in early childhood, affected individuals may have relatively large benign tumors that consist of bundles of nerves. Individuals with NF-1 may also develop benign tumor-like nodules of the colored regions of the eyes or tumors of the optic nerves, which transmit nerve impulses from the innermost, nerve-rich membrane of the eyes (retinas) to the brain. More rarely, affected individuals may develop certain malignant tumors.

NF-1 is caused by mutations of a relatively large gene. The gene regulates the production of a protein known as *neurofibromin.* This can cause problems in a child's function owing to fatigue resulting from malignant tumors and limitations resulting from visual difficulties.

Precautions

Impact on Performance Skills

The term *neurofibromatosis* is sometimes used to describe NF-1 as well as a second, distinct form of NF (NF-2). NF-2 is an autosomal dominant disorder that is primarily characterized by benign tumors of both acoustic nerves, leading to progressive hearing loss. The auditory nerves transmit nerve impulses from the inner ear to the brain.

NF-1 may be characterized by unusual largeness of the head and relatively short stature. Additional abnormalities may also be present, such as episodes of brain seizures; learning disabilities; speech difficulties; abnormally increased activity; and skeletal malformations, including scoliosis, bowing of the lower legs, and improper development of certain bones. In individuals with NF-1, associated symptoms and findings may vary greatly in range and severity from case to case. Most people with NF-1 have normal intelligence, but learning disabilities appear in some children.

Both types of neurofibromatosis can affect motor skills, process skills, and communication and interaction skills.

Impact on Client Factors (Body Functions and Structures)

NF can cause skin changes, bone deformities, and other problems. It can also cause developmental abnormalities and learning disabilities. Symptoms vary greatly and generally get worse over time. In-home and classroom adaptations may be necessary if a child has learning difficulties.

Evaluation

- Clinical observations
- Client and caregiver interview
- Checklists or observation of community, school, and home child-environment fit

Suggested Assessment Tools

- Alberta Infant Motor Scale (AIMS)
- Assessment of Motor and Process Skills (AMPS)
- Bayley Scales of Infant Development (BSID)
- Bruininks-Oseretsky Test of Motor Proficiency (BOT-2)
- Canadian Occupational Performance Measure (COPM)
- Child Occupational Self Assessment (COSA)
- Denver Developmental Screening Test (DDST)
- Hawaii Early Learning Profile (HELP)
- Home Observation and Measurement of the Environment (HOME)
- Infant/Toddler Sensory Profile

N

- Movement Assessment for Infants (MAI)
- Pediatric Evaluation of Disability Inventory (PEDI)
- School Function Assessment (SFA)
- School Setting Interview (SSI)
- Short Child Occupational Profile (SCOPE)
- Toddler and Infant Motor Evaluation (TIME)
- Wee FIM

INTERVENTIONS

- Home, community, and classroom modifications and adaptations
- Positioning
- Behavior modification in consultation with school psychologist or trained behavior therapist

Case Example

Tomas is a 10-year-old with NF-1. He has been having trouble in his class due to being hyperactive as well as exhibiting signs of a learning disability. The school occupational therapist has been asked to assess Tomas to determine the specific client-environment needs. ❖

WEB RESOURCES

Neurofibromatosis, Inc.
www.nfinc.org

Children's Tumor Foundation
www.ctf.org

March of Dimes
www.marchofdimes.com/newsletters/February_2004.asp

FURTHER READING

Evans DG, Baser ME, O'Reilly B, et al: Management of the patient and family with neurofibromatosis 2: a consensus conference statement, *Br J Neurosurg* 19:5, 2005.

Furlong W, Barr RD, Feeny D, Yandow S: Patient-focused measures of functional health status and health-related quality of life in pediatric orthopedics: a case study in measurement selection, *Health Qual Life Outcomes* 3:3, 2005.

North K, Joy P, Yuille D, et al: Specific learning disability in children with neurofibromatosis type 1: significance of MRI abnormalities, *Neurology* 44:878, 1994.

N

61

❖

Nystagmus

Epidemiology

Nystagmus consists of involuntary, rhythmic, repeated oscillations of one or both eyes, in any or all fields of gaze. Movements may be pendular or jerky and may be horizontal, vertical, oblique, rotary, circular, or any combination of these.

Congenital Nystagmus

Congenital nystagmus manifests as oscillating eye movements by 2 to 3 months of age. The eyes usually move in a horizontal direction in a swinging fashion. Vision is typically reduced and sometimes poor. The cause of congenital nystagmus is frequently unknown.

Spasmus Nutans

Spasmus nutans manifests between 6 months and 3 years of age and resolves spontaneously between 2 and 8 years of age. Patients with spasmus nutans have head nodding and a head turn, and the eyes may move in any direction. This condition does not require any treatment.

Acquired Nystagmus

Acquired nystagmus manifests in later childhood or adulthood. Acquired nystagmus may be categorized as unknown; inherited; secondary to central nervous system disorders,

N

metabolic disorders, or toxicity from alcohol and drugs; or physiologic.

Impact on Performance Skills

Children with nystagmus may experience delays in process skills such as the following:

- Knowledge
- Organization of space and objects
- Adaptation

Typically children with nystagmus will not demonstrate delays in motor or communication and interaction skills.

Impact on Client Factors (Body Functions and Structures)

The defect is classified according to the position of the eyes when it occurs. Grade I occurs only when the eyes are directed toward the fast component; grade II occurs when the eyes are also in their primary position; grade III occurs even when the eyes are directed toward the slow component. Reduced acuity is caused by the inability to maintain steady fixation. This can potentially affect a child's process skills.

Precautions

Impact on Performance Skills

Congenital nystagmus is more common than acquired nystagmus. It is usually mild, does not change in severity, and is not associated with any other disorder. A less common cause of acquired nystagmus is disease or injury of the central nervous system. This can potentially cause problems in learning if severe enough. Visual acuity may be less than 20/20. Surgery may improve visual acuity.

Impact on Client Factors (Body Functions and Structures)

Children with nystagmus, who may tend to lose their place in beginning reading instruction, may be helped through the use of a typoscope (card with a rectangular hole, to view one word or line at a time) or an underliner (card or strip of paper to "underline" the line being read). As children with nystagmus mature, they seem to need these support devices less often.

Evaluation

- Clinical observations
- Interview of client, family, teachers
- Infant or child environment in home, community, and school

Suggested Assessment Tools

- Balcones Sensory Integration Screening Kit
- Beery-Butenica Developmental Test of Visual-Motor Integration, Fourth Edition
- Developmental Test of Visual Perception, Second Edition (DTVP-2)
- Visual Acuity

INTERVENTIONS

- Environmental accommodations and modifications
- Task modifications and accommodations

Case Example

Tamar is a 7-year-old who has trouble following along when there is a reading assignment in her class. The occupational therapist has adapted the environment and offered the teacher suggestions for adapting tasks to address Tamar's needs. ❖

WEB RESOURCES

American Nystagmus Network
www.nystagmus.org

Nystagmus Network
www.nystagmusnet.org

N

FURTHER READING

Ottenbacher K: Patterns of postrotary nystagmus in three learning-disabled children, *Am J Occup Ther* 36:657, 1982.

Ottenbacher K, Watson PJ, Short MA, Biderman MD: Nystagmus and ocular fixation difficulties in learning-disabled children, *Am J Occup Ther* 33:717, 1979.

N

62

❖

Obesity

Epidemiology

Obesity is the condition of having too much body fat. It is different from being overweight, which means weighing too much. Both terms mean that a child's weight is greater than what is considered healthy for his or her height.

Impact on Performance Skills

Children with obesity may experience delays in motor skills such as the following:

- Posture
- Mobility
- Coordination
- Strength and effort
- Energy

Typically children with obesity will not demonstrate delays in process or communication and interaction skills.

Impact on Client Factors (Body Functions and Structures)

Most overweight young people have at least one additional risk factor for heart disease. Overweight young people are more likely than children of normal weight to become overweight or obese adults. This can limit participation in motor activities due to low energy and fatigue.

O

Precautions

Impact on Performance Skills

Children who are overweight are at greater risk for bone and joint problems, sleep apnea, and social and psychologic problems such as stigmatization and poor self-esteem. This can be exhibited through the child's limited motor performance.

Impact on Client Factors (Body Functions and Structures)

If a weight-loss program is necessary, the whole family needs to be involved so the child does not feel singled out.

Evaluation

- Observation
- Leisure interests
- Interview

Suggested Assessment Tools

- Canadian Occupational Performance Measure (COPM)
- Child Occupational Self Assessment (COSA)
- Children's Assessment of Participation and Enjoyment (CAPE)
- Leisure Boredom Scale (LBS)
- Leisure Competence Measure
- Leisure Diagnostic Battery
- Leisure Satisfaction Scale
- Pediatric Interest Profile (PIP)
- Pediatric Volitional Questionnaire (PVQ)
- Preferences for Activities of Children (PAC)
- Short Child Occupational Profile (SCOPE)

INTERVENTIONS

- Encourage healthy eating by discussing the nutritional value of fruits and vegetables and the problems with having a large intake of sodas and high-calorie, high-fat snack foods.
- Involve the family in changing a child's diet and activity level in the home.
- Explore active leisure options.

o

Case Example

Lynda is a 12-year-old with a medical diagnosis of obesity. She typically spends her free time watching TV and playing computer games. The occupational therapist has been consulting with Lynda and her family to identify new active leisure pastimes that interest Lynda. ❖

WEB RESOURCE

American Academy of Pediatrics
www.aap.orgobesity

FURTHER READING

Blanchard SA: AOTA's statement on obesity, *Am J Occup Ther* 60:680, 2006.

Roblin L: Childhood obesity: food, nutrient, and eating-habit trends and influences, *Appl Physiol Nutr Metab* 32:635, 2007.

Shaw J: Epidemiology of childhood type 2 diabetes and obesity, *Pediatr Diabetes* 8(Suppl 9):17, 2007.

Styles JL, Meier A, Sutherland LA, Campbell MK: Parents' and caregivers' concerns about obesity in young children: a qualitative study, *Fam Community Health* 30:279, 2007.

Wilson LF: Adolescents' attitudes about obesity and what they want in obesity prevention programs, *J Sch Nurs* 23:229, 2007.

63

❖

Oppositional Defiant Disorder

Epidemiology

Oppositional defiant disorder (ODD) is characterized by consistent disobedience or hostile or defiant behavior toward authority figures. The pattern of behavior must last for more than 6 months and must be compared with the behaviors of other children of the same age. Some signs and symptoms include the following behaviors:

- Is argumentative
- Easily loses temper
- Blames others for own mistakes
- Has difficulty making friends or sustaining friendships
- Is often angry
- Uses vindictive behavior toward others
- Is easily annoyed
- Defies adults and authority figures
- Is often in trouble in school

If a child is a danger to himself or herself or to others, hospitalization may be necessary.

Impact on Performance Skills

Children with ODD may experience problems with communication and interaction skills such as the following:

O

- Physicality
- Information exchange
- Relations

Children with ODD will not demonstrate problems with motor skills or process skills.

Impact on Client Factors (Body Functions and Structures)

ODD is manifested through a child's behaviors and personality. Affected children are defiant, and this affects ability to engage in tasks, especially when an authority figure such as a teacher in a classroom is involved.

Precautions
Impact on Performance Skills

ODD is not usually the only issue that a child is experiencing. It may be necessary to complete a battery of evaluations to determine if there are additional existing conditions. Attention deficit and hyperactivity disorder (ADHD), anxiety disorders, and mood disorders such as depression and bipolar disorder are a few conditions that may coexist with ODD. It is important to treat all conditions a child is facing in order to improve participation.

Impact on Client Factors (Body Functions and Structures)

Children with ODD are at risk for getting in trouble at school, in the home, and in the community owing to their negative behavior. This can affect socialization and self-esteem.

Evaluation
- Interviews with child and family
- Environmental observations
- Social skills

Suggested Assessment Tools

- Bay Area Functional Performance Evaluation (BaFPE)
- Behavior Assessment Rating Scale (BASC)
- Child Behavior Checklist (CBCL)
- Early Coping Inventory
- Interest Checklist/NPI Interest Checklist
- Occupational Circumstances Assessment Interview and Rating Scale (OCAIRS)
- Occupational Performance History Interview (Version 2) (OPHI-2)
- Self-Assessment of Occupational Functioning (SAOF)
- Social Skills Rating System

INTERVENTIONS

- Behavior modification program in consultation with the school psychologist or a trained behavior therapist
- Leisure exploration

Case Example

Bobby is a 15-year-old with ODD. He has been in trouble at school for outbursts in class and typically is sent to in-school suspension. The occupational therapist has been asked to develop a behavior modification program with the school psychologist to implement in the class. ❖

WEB RESOURCES

American Academy of Childhood and Adolescent Psychiatry
http://aacap.org

Conductdisorders.com
www.conductdisorders.com

O

FURTHER READING

Keen DV: Conduct disorders and us: from heart sink to heart warming? *Arch Dis Child* 92:838, 2007.

Lavigne JV, Lebailly SA, Gouze KR, et al: Treating oppositional defiant disorder in primary care: a comparison of three models, *J Pediatr Psychol* Oct 23, 2007 [Epub ahead of print].

64

❖

Osteogenesis Imperfecta

Epidemiology

Osteogenesis imperfecta (OI), also known as *brittle bone disease,* is an inherited condition that results from an abnormality in type I collagen in the body. Type I collagen fibers are found in bones, tendons, the skin, and the eyes. OI usually begins either in utero or in infancy.

Almost all individuals with OI have fragile bones that break easily. There are eight types of OI.

Impact on Performance Skills

Children with OI may experience delays in motor skills such as the following:

- Posture
- Mobility
- Strength and effort

Children with OI may experience delays in communication and interaction skills such as the following:

- Physicality

Children with OI will not demonstrate delays in process skills.

Impact on Client Factors (Body Functions and Structures)

Long periods of immobilization can decrease mobility and increase the risk of future fractures, making it important to

O

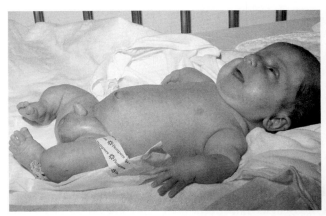

Osteogenesis imperfecta type II. This infant was born with multiple fractures and limb deformities. (From Zitelli BJ, Davis HW: *Atlas of pediatric physical diagnosis,* ed 5, St Louis, 2007, Mosby.)

encourage movement and weight bearing as soon as possible after a fracture.

Precautions

Impact on Performance Skills

OI can range from mild to severe, and symptoms vary from child to child. A person may have just a few or as many as several hundred fractures in a lifetime. There is no cure, but symptoms can be managed. This results in limitations in motor activity and affects the needs a child has in positioning in the environment.

Impact on Client Factors (Body Functions and Structures)

Most treatment, even of fractures, will be nonsurgical. Casting, bracing, or splinting a fracture is necessary to immobilize the bone so that healing can occur. This limits participation, which makes it important to address this need with the child, family, and context that the child is in.

Evaluation

- Clinical observation
- Parent or caregiver interview
- Child interview
- Community, home, and school observation

Suggested Assessment Tools

- Canadian Occupational Performance Measure (COPM)
- Child Occupational Self Assessment (COSA)
- Children's Assessment of Participation and Enjoyment (CAPE)
- Classroom Observation Guide
- Home Observation and Measurement of the Environment (HOME)
- Klein-Bell Activities of Daily Living Scale
- Leisure Satisfaction Scale
- Occupational Circumstances Assessment Interview and Rating Scale (OCAIRS)
- Occupational Performance History Interview (Version 2) (OPHI-2)
- Pediatric Evaluation of Disability Inventory (PEDI)
- Self Assessment of Occupational Functioning (SAOF)
- Short Child Occupational Profile (SCOPE)

INTERVENTIONS

- Positioning
- Task modification and adaptation
- Environment modification and adaptation
- Exercise program
- Family education in child care to limit fractures

O

*Case Example*_____

Zach, an 8-month-old infant, has OI. The occupational therapist has been working with Zach's mother to identify his positioning needs in relation to his car seat, stroller, bed, and highchair to limit fractures. ❖

WEB RESOURCE

Osteogenesis Imperfecta Foundation
www.oif.orgsite/PageServer

FURTHER READING

Binder H, Conway A, Gerber LH: Rehabilitation approaches to children with osteogenesis imperfecta: a ten-year experience, *Arch Phys Med Rehabil* 74:386, 1993.

Martin E, Shapiro JR: Osteogenesis imperfecta: epidemiology and pathophysiology, *Curr Osteoporos Rep* 5:91, 2007.

Tainmont J: History of osteogenesis imperfecta or brittle bone disease: a few stops on a road 3000 years long, *B-ENT* 3:157, 2007.

65

❖

Patau's Syndrome (Trisomy 13)

Epidemiology

Trisomy 13 is a syndrome associated with the presence of a third chromosome (an extra number 13). Trisomy 13 is a syndrome with multiple abnormalities, many of which are not compatible with life. Most children with trisomy 13 die in the first month.

Trisomy 13 can be diagnosed prenatally. Because of the severity of congenital defects, life-sustaining procedures are generally not attempted.

Impact on Performance Skills

Children with trisomy 13 may experience delays in motor skills such as the following:
- Mobility
- Coordination
- Strength and effort
- Energy

Children with trisomy 13 may experience delays in process skills such as the following:
- Energy
- Knowledge
- Temporal organization
- Adaptation

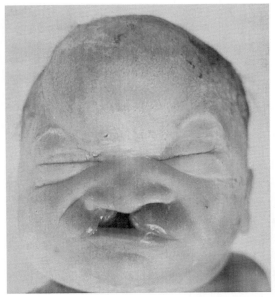

Trisomy 13. (From Zitelli BJ, Davis HW: *Atlas of pediatric physical diagnosis,* ed 5, St Louis, 2007, Mosby.)

Children with trisomy 13 may experience delays in communication and interaction skills such as the following:
- Physicality
- Relations

Impact on Client Factors (Body Functions and Structures)

Trisomy 13 is associated with multiple abnormalities, including defects of the brain that lead to seizures, apnea, deafness, and eye abnormalities. This affects motor function, sensory processing, and visual processing.

Precautions

Impact on Performance Skills

Children with trisomy 13 have small eyes with deficits in the iris and can have a cleft lip and palate as well as low-set ears. Many children also have congenital heart disease as well as hernias and genital abnormalities. Magnetic resonance imaging (MRI) or computed tomography (CT) scans of the head may reveal a structural abnormality of the brain, called *holoprosencephaly,* in which the two cerebral hemispheres are fused. Complications begin almost immediately. The condition leads to problems with breathing, deafness, vision problems, feeding problems, seizures, and heart failure.

Impact on Client Factors (Body Functions and Structures)

Children with trisomy 13 can exhibit the following:

- Severe intellectual disabilities
- Seizures
- Microcephaly
- Scalp defects (absent skin)
- Small eyes
- Cleft lip and/or palate
- Eyes close set (eyes may actually fuse together into one)
- Iris defects
- Pinna abnormalities and low-set ears
- Simian crease
- Extra digits
- Hernias
- Undescended testicle
- Hypotonia
- Micrognathia
- Skeletal (limb) abnormalities

Gastrointestinal x-ray or ultrasound examination may reveal abnormal rotation of the internal organs.

Evaluation

- Parent or caregiver interview
- Clinical observation

Suggested Assessment Tools

- Alberta Infant Motor Scale (AIMS)
- Erhardt Developmental Prehension Assessment (EDPA)
- Erhardt Developmental Vision Assessment, Revised (EDVA)
- Gross Motor Function Measure (GMFM)
- Hawaii Early Learning Profile (HELP)
- Home Observation and Measurement of the Environment (HOME)
- Pediatric Evaluation of Disability Inventory (PEDI)
- Short Child Occupational Profile (SCOPE)
- Toddler and Infant Motor Evaluation (TIME)
- WeeFIM

INTERVENTIONS

- Positioning
- Caregiver training and education

Case Example

Shoshanna is a newborn who has been diagnosed with trisomy 13. The occupational therapist has received an order to evaluate and treat. The occupational therapist decides to use assessments to gather baseline developmental data. ❖

WEB RESOURCES

Genetics Home Reference
http://ghr.nlm.nih.gov/condition=trisomy13

National Organization for Rare Disorders
www.rarediseases.orgsearch/rdbdetail_abstract.html?disname=Trisomy%2013%20Syndrome

March of Dimes
www.marchofdimes.com

The Arc (a national organization on mental retardation)
www.thearc.org

Support Organization for Trisomy 18, 13, and Related Disorders (SOFT)
www.trisomy.org

Living with Trisomy 13
www.livingwithtrisomy13.org

FURTHER READING

Singh KS: Trisomy 13 (Patau's syndrome): a rare case of survival into adulthood, *J Ment Defic Res* 34(Pt 1):91, 1990.

66

❖

Periventricular Leukomalacia

Epidemiology

Periventricular leukomalacia (PVL) is a type of brain injury in which small areas of brain tissue around fluid-filled areas of the brain die. The tissue death creates "holes" in the brain. PVL is frequently associated with neurologic and developmental problems in growing babies, usually during the first to second year of life.

There is no treatment for PVL. The baby's heart, lung, intestine, and kidney functions will be monitored and treated so they remain as normal as possible.

A major cause is thought to be poor blood flow to the area around the ventricles of the brain, which is fragile and prone to injury. Infection around the time of delivery may play a role in causing PVL.

Impact on Performance Skills

Children with PVL may experience delays in motor skills such as the following:

- Posture
- Mobility
- Coordination
- Strength and effort
- Energy

Children with PVL may experience delays in process skills such as the following:

- Energy
- Knowledge
- Temporal organization
- Organization of space and objects
- Adaptation

Children with PVL may experience delays in communication and interaction skills such as the following:

- Physicality
- Information exchange

Impact on Client Factors (Body Functions and Structures)

Babies with PVL are at risk for significant neurologic problems, especially those that involve motor skills such as sitting, crawling, walking, and moving the arms.

Precautions

Impact on Performance Skills

A baby diagnosed with PVL should be monitored for a variety of developmental delays. These delays can affect motor function, process skills, and communication and interaction, which can limit participation in daily activities.

Impact on Client Factors (Body Functions and Structures)

The more premature and sick a baby is, the higher the risk for PVL. If a baby has PVL, he or she will have limitations in a variety of skills and in most of the contexts he or she is in.

Evaluation

- Clinical observations
- Home, community, and school environment observations
- Parent or caregiver interview

Suggested Assessment Tools

- Alberta Infant Motor Scale (AIMS)
- Assessment of Motor and Process Skills (AMPS)

- Bayley Scale of Infant Development
- Canadian Occupational Performance Measure (COPM)
- DeGangi-Berk Test of Sensory Integration (TSI)
- Erhardt Developmental Prehension Assessment (EDPA)
- Home Observation and Measurement of the Environment (HOME)
- Infant/Toddler Sensory Profile
- Movement Assessment for Infants (MAI)
- Peabody Developmental Motor Scales 2, Revised (PDMS-2)
- Pediatric Evaluation of Disability Inventory (PEDI)
- Short Child Occupational Profile (SCOPE)
- Toddler and Infant Motor Evaluation (TIME)

INTERVENTIONS

- Task modification and adaptation
- Environment modification and adaptation
- Positioning
- Family education and home program

Case Example

Vince is a 2-year-old with PVL. The occupational therapist from early intervention provides adapted toys for Vince to play with owing to his motor delays. The occupational therapist also has made recommendations for environmental modifications within the home to accommodate Vince. ⋄

WEB RESOURCE

National Institute of Neurological Disorders and Stroke
**www.ninds.nih.gov/disorders/periventricular_leukomalacia/
periventricular_leukomalacia.htm**

FURTHER READING

Pagliano E, Fedrizzi E, Erbetta A, et al: Cognitive profiles and visuoperceptual abilities in preterm and term spastic diplegic children with periventricular leukomalacia, *J Child Neurol* 22:282, 2007.

Pierson CR, Folkerth RD, Billiards SS, et al: Gray matter injury associated with periventricular leukomalacia in the premature infant, *Acta Neuropathol* 114:619, 2007.

Vergani P, Locatelli A, Doria V, et al: Intraventricular hemorrhage and periventricular leukomalacia in preterm infants, *Obstet Gynecol* 104:225, 2004.

P

67

❖

Persistent Pulmonary Hypertension

Epidemiology

Persistent pulmonary hypertension of the newborn (PPHN) is also known as *persistent fetal circulation*. This is a condition in which a newborn baby's circulation changes back to the circulation of a fetus, where much of the blood flow bypasses the lungs. It occurs most often in full-term or postterm babies after a difficult birth or from birth asphyxia (a condition that results from too little oxygen). The symptoms of PPHN may resemble those of other conditions or medical problems.

When a baby has lowered oxygen levels or difficulty breathing at birth, these changes may not occur and the baby's circulation returns back to the fetal system, with blood directed away from the lungs. The lung pressure stays high. That is why this condition is called *persistent pulmonary hypertension*. Treatment of PPHN is aimed at increasing the oxygen to the rest of the body systems.

Impact on Performance Skills

Children with PPHN may experience delays in motor skills such as the following:

- Posture
- Mobility
- Coordination

P

- Strength and effort
- Energy

Children with PPHN may experience delays in process skills such as the following:

- Energy
- Knowledge
- Temporal organization
- Organization of space and objects
- Adaptation

Children with PPHN may experience delays in communication and interaction skills such as the following:

- Physicality
- Information exchange
- Relations

Impact on Client Factors (Body Functions and Structures)

Long-term health problems may be related to damage from lowered oxygen in the body, and this can result in neurologic impairments, which can affect motor skills.

Precautions

Impact on Performance Skills

Children with PPHN have difficulties developing motor skills to participate in daily and play activities.

Impact on Client Factors (Body Functions and Structures)

The following are the most common signs of PPHN. However, each baby may manifest signs differently.

- Baby appears ill at delivery or in first hours after birth
- Cyanosis (blue coloring)
- Rapid breathing
- Rapid heart rate
- Low blood oxygen levels while receiving 100% oxygen

These all lead to developmental delays in motor, process, and communication and interaction skills. There is also the potential for sensory disorders.

Evaluation
- Clinical observations
- Parent or caregiver interview
- Infant or child-environment fit

Suggested Assessment Tools
- Alberta Infant Motor Scale (AIMS)
- Denver Developmental Screening Test (DDST)
- Early Coping Inventory
- Hawaii Early Learning Profile (HELP)
- Home Observation and Measurement of the Environment (HOME)
- Infant/Toddler Sensory Profile
- Movement Assessment for Infants (MAI)
- Peabody Developmental Motor Scales 2, Revised (PDMS-2)
- Pediatric Evaluation of Disability Inventory (PEDI)
- Short Child Occupational Profile (SCOPE)
- Vineland Adaptive Behavior Scales Revised (VABS)
- WeeFIM

INTERVENTIONS
- Task modification and adaptation
- Environment accommodation and adaptation
- Positioning
- Parent or caregiver education

Case Example
Mohammad, a newborn, has been diagnosed with PPHN. The occupational therapist has been working on positioning and providing suggestions for adapting his environment based on his motor delays due to PPHN. ❖

P

WEB RESOURCES

Persistent Pulmonary Hypertension of Newborns
**www.pph-newborn.org?gaw-prinew&gclid=
COGsuIuuy4wCFRE9VAodrD0Pag**

Medicineworld.org
**http://medicineworld.orgcancer/lead/10-2006/babies-with-persistent-
pulmonary-hypertension.html**

FURTHER READING

Donti A, Formigari R, Ragni L, et al: Pulmonary arterial hypertension in the pediatric age, *J Cardiovasc Med (Hagerstown)* 8:72, 2007.

Hernández-Díaz S, Van Marter LJ, Werler MM, et al: Risk factors for persistent pulmonary hypertension of the newborn, *Pediatrics* 120:e272, 2007.

Verklan MT: Persistent pulmonary hypertension of the newborn: not a honeymoon anymore, *J Perinat Neonatal Nurs* 20:108, 2006.

68

❖

Phenylketonuria

Epidemiology

Phenylketonuria (PKU) is a genetic disorder in which the body is unable to process part of a protein called *phenylalanine* (Phe). Phe is found in almost all foods.

Impact on Performance Skills

Children with PKU may experience delays in motor skills such as the following:

- Posture
- Mobility
- Coordination
- Strength and effort
- Energy

Children with PKU may experience delays in process skills such as the following:

- Energy
- Knowledge
- Temporal organization
- Organization of space and objects
- Adaptation

Children with PKU may experience delays in communication and interaction skills such as the following:

- Physicality
- Information exchange
- Relations

Impact on Client Factors (Body Functions and Structures)

If the Phe level gets too high, it can damage the brain and cause severe intellectual disabilities. This can affect a child's functioning in all areas and in a variety of situations.

Precautions

Impact on Performance Skills

The best treatment for PKU is a diet of low-protein foods. There are special formulas for newborns. For older children and adults, the diet includes many fruits and vegetables. It also includes some low-protein breads, pastas, and cereals. Parent education about the dietary needs of infants with PKU is necessary. If an infant has PKU and there is brain damage, there may be issues with motor, process, and communication and interaction skills.

Impact on Client Factors (Body Functions and Structures)

Babies who get on a special diet soon after they are born develop normally. Many have no signs of PKU. It is important that they stay on the diet for the rest of their lives.

Evaluation

- Clinical observation
- Parent or caregiver interview
- Infant or child environment fit

Suggested Assessment Tools

- Alberta Infant Motor Scale (AIMS)
- Early Coping Inventory
- Erhardt Developmental Prehension Assessment (EDPA)
- Erhardt Developmental Vision Assessment, Revised (EVDA)
- Hawaii Early Learning Profile (HELP)
- Home Observation and Measurement of the Environment (HOME)

P

- Infant/Toddler Sensory Profile
- Movement Assessment for Infants (MAI)
- Peabody Developmental Motor Scales 2, Revised (PDMS-2)
- Pediatric Evaluation of Disability Inventory (PEDI)
- Short Child Occupational Profile (SCOPE)
- Toddler and Infant Motor Evaluation (TIME)
- Vineland Adaptive Behavior Scales, Revised (VABS)
- WeeFIM

INTERVENTIONS

- Positioning
- Parent or caregiver training
- Environment modification and adaptation
- Sensory modulation

Case Example

Charles, a 6-month-old, has been diagnosed with PKU. He has limited movement and postural control. The occupational therapist is working with his family to address his motor delays through positioning and appropriate play activities. ❖

WEB RESOURCES

National PKU News
www.pkunews.org

March of Dimes
www.marchofdimes.com/pnhec/4439_1219.asp

National Organization for Rare Disorders
www.rarediseases.orgsearch/rdbdetail_abstract.html?disname= Phenylketonuria

FURTHER READING

Bilginsoy C, Waitzman N, Leonard CO, Ernst SL: Living with phenylketon-uria: perspectives of patients and their families, *J Inherit Metab Dis* 28:639, 2005.

Giovannini M, Riva E, Salvatici E, et al: Treating phenylketonuria: a single centre experience, *J Int Med Res* 35(6):742-752, 2007.

Phenylketonuria (PKU): screening and management, *NIH Consens Statement* 17:1, 2000.

69

❖

Pica

Epidemiology

Pica is a pattern of eating nonfood materials (such as dirt or paper). This pattern should last at least 1 month to fit the diagnosis of pica. Pica is seen more in young children than in adults, with a number of children aged 1 to 6 exhibiting these behaviors.

Impact on Performance Skills

Children with pica may experience delays in motor skills such as the following:
- Posture
- Mobility
- Coordination
- Strength and effort
- Energy

Children with pica will not have delays in process or communication and interaction skills.

Impact on Client Factors (Body Functions and Structures)

Treatment success varies. In many cases the disorder lasts several months and then disappears on its own. In some cases it may continue into the teen years or adulthood, particularly when associated with developmental disorders.

Complications that can occur with pica include the following:

P

- Malnutrition
- Lead toxicity
- Infection
- Bezoar (a hardened mass of the substance in the stomach)
- Intestinal obstruction

There is no specific prevention. Adequate nutrition may be helpful.

Precautions

Impact on Performance Skills

It is important to address any nutritional deficiencies or other medical problems, such as lead toxicity.

Medications may help reduce the abnormal eating behavior if pica occurs as part of a developmental disorder such as mental retardation. It is also important to address any limitations in motor skills or process skills resulting from this disorder.

Impact on Client Factors (Body Functions and Structures)

There is no single test that confirms pica, but because pica is associated with abnormal nutrient levels and in some cases malnutrition, blood levels of iron and zinc should be tested. Nutrition and behavior will need to be addressed in addition to helping the family to cope with this disorder.

Evaluation

- Clinical observation
- Parent or caregiver interview
- Infant or child environment fit

Suggested Assessment Tools

- Bayley Scale of Infant Development (BSID)
- Denver Developmental Screening Test (DDST)

P

- Early Coping Inventory
- Home Observation and Measurement of the Environment (HOME)
- Infant/Toddler Sensory Profile
- Short Child Occupational Profile (SCOPE)

INTERVENTIONS

- Parent or caregiver education
- Environment modification and adaptation
- Sensory modulation
- Feeding

Case Example

Shanta is a 10-year-old being treated for pica. An occupational therapist has been asked to consult and co-treat with a speech language pathologist to address possible sensory aversion issues with feeding. ❖

WEB RESOURCES

Healthline
**www.healthline.com/search?q1=pica&imuId=2791241&utm_medium=
google&utm_source=eating_disorders&utm_campaign=
serp&utm_term=pica**

Medscape Today
www.medscape.com/viewarticle/405804_7

PsychNet-UK
www.psychnet-uk.com/dsm_iv/pica_disorder.htm

FURTHER READING

Boukthir S: Does your child have pica? *Acta Gastroenterol Belg* 70:245, 2007.

Fotoulaki M, Panagopoulou P, Efstratiou I, Nousia-Arvanitakis S: Pitfalls in the approach to pica, *Eur J Pediatr* 166:623, 2007.

Kern L, Starosta K, Adelman BE: Reducing pica by teaching children to exchange inedible items for edibles, *Behav Modif* 30:135, 2006.

Rose EA, Porcerelli JH, Neale AV: Pica: common but commonly missed, *J Am Board Fam Pract* 13:353, 2000.

70

❖

Posttraumatic Stress Disorder

Epidemiology

Posttraumatic stress disorder (PTSD) is one of only a few mental disorders that are triggered by a disturbing outside event, quite unlike most other psychiatric disorders. Events that might cause PTSD include rape, physical abuse, an airplane or car crash, war, or other traumatic events. For most children, PTSD starts about 3 months after the event. However, sometimes signs of PTSD show up years later.

Impact on Performance Skills

Children with PTSD may experience delays in motor skills such as the following:
- Energy

Children with PTSD may experience delays in process skills such as the following:
- Energy
- Knowledge
- Temporal organization
- Organization of space and objects
- Adaptation

Children with PTSD may experience delays in communication and interaction skills such as the following:

P

- Physicality
- Information exchange
- Relations

Impact on Client Factors (Body Functions and Structures)

The worse the trauma, the more likely a child will develop PTSD, and the worse the symptoms will be. Many children are so severely affected that they are unable to do schoolwork, have trouble with relationships and friendships, and have great difficulty interacting with others.

Precautions

Impact on Performance Skills

Often, children have the following reactions when PTSD occurs:

- Feeling like the event is happening again
- Trouble sleeping or nightmares
- Not feeling close to people
- Becoming easily angered
- Feeling guilty because others died when the child lived

Impact on Client Factors (Body Functions and Structures)

It is difficult to adapt to life after a traumatic event. PTSD reflects a state of being unable to "stop remembering" the event, to the point that it affects daily life. Many children experience individual traumatic events, such as car and airplane accidents to sexual assault, or they can experience other events such as natural disasters or war.

Evaluation

- Clinical observations
- Client interview
- Parent or caregiver interview
- Child-environment fit

P

Suggested Assessment Tools
- Child Behavior Checklist (CBCL)
- Coping Inventory
- Occupational Circumstances Assessment Interview and Rating Scale (OCAIRS)
- Occupational Performance History Interview (Version 2) (OPHI-2)
- Self-Assessment of Occupational Functioning (SAOF)
- Short Child Occupational Profile (SCOPE)

INTERVENTIONS
- Environment accommodations and adaptations
- Task modifications and adaptations
- Leisure interests

Case Example

Rhonda is 15 years old and is experiencing PTSD. She is having difficulty focusing on tasks and attending to course work in school. The occupational therapist is working with Rhonda and the school psychologist to help modify Rhonda's environment so she can function at an optimal level. ❖

WEB RESOURCES
American Academy of Family Physicians
http://familydoctor.orgonline/famdocen/home/common/mentalhealth/anxiety/624.html

National Center for PTSD
http://ncptsd.va.gov/ncmain/ncdocs/fact_shts/fs_what_can_i_do.html

PTSD Alliance
www.ptsdalliance.org

FURTHER READING
Adler-Nevo G, Manassis K: Psychosocial treatment of pediatric posttraumatic stress disorder: the neglected field of single-incident trauma, *Depress Anxiety* 22:177, 2005.

De Bellis MD, Van Dillen T: Childhood post-traumatic stress disorder: an overview, *Child Adolesc Psychiatr Clin N Am* 14:745, 2005.

Mulvihill D: Nursing care of children after a traumatic incident, *Issues Compr Pediatr Nurs* 30:15, 2007.

Simó-Algado S, Mehta N, Kronenberg F, et al: Occupational therapy intervention with children survivors of war, *Can J Occup Ther* 69:205, 2002.

Zehnder D, Prchal A, Vollrath M, Landolt MA: Prospective study of the effectiveness of coping in pediatric patients, *Child Psychiatry Hum Dev* 36:351, 2006.

71

❖

Pneumonia

Epidemiology

Pneumonia is an inflammation of the lungs caused by an infection. Many different organisms can cause it, including bacteria, viruses, and fungi. Pneumonia is a common illness; it can range from mild to severe and can even be fatal. The severity depends on the type of organism causing the pneumonia, as well as the patient's age and underlying health.

Bacterial pneumonias tend to be the most serious and in adults are the most common type of pneumonia.

Respiratory viruses are the most common causes of pneumonia in young children, peaking between the ages of 2 and 3.

Impact on Performance Skills

Children with pneumonia may experience delays in motor skills such as the following:

- Mobility
- Strength and effort
- Energy

Children with pneumonia may experience delays in process skills such as the following:

- Energy

Children with pneumonia will not have delays in communication and interaction skills.

P

Impact on Client Factors (Body Functions and Structures)

Children with pneumonia may be working hard to breathe or may be breathing fast. They need to get lots of rest and drink plenty of fluids to help loosen secretions; if fever is present, it must be controlled.

If a child is admitted to the hospital, the treatment can include respiratory therapy to assist with secretions. Steroids may be used to reduce wheezing if a child has an underlying lung disease. Some children respond to treatment within the first 2 weeks, whereas others may fail to respond and can die from respiratory failure.

Precautions

Impact on Performance Skills

Empyemata or lung abscesses are infrequent, but serious, complications of pneumonia. They occur when pockets of pus form around or inside the lung. These may sometimes require surgical drainage. This can leave a child weak and fatigued. This will limit motor activities and possibly affect a child's motor skills owing to muscle weakness from muscle atrophy.

Impact on Client Factors (Body Functions and Structures)

Signs and symptoms of pneumonia typically seen in children are as follows:
  • Cough with greenish or yellow mucus
  • Occasional bloody sputum
  • Fever with shaking chills
  • Sharp or stabbing chest pain worsened by deep breathing or coughing
  • Rapid, shallow breathing
  • Shortness of breath
Pneumonia can lead to difficulties for children with participation in a variety of activities owing to weakness and fatigue.

P

Evaluation
- Clinical observations
- Child-environment fit

Suggested Assessment Tools
- Canadian Occupational Performance Measure (COPM)
- Short Child Occupational Profile (SCOPE)
- WeeFIM

INTERVENTIONS
- Environment modification and adaptation
- Task modification and adaptation
- Energy conservation

Case Example

Jerome, a 7-year-old, has been admitted to the hospital because of pneumonia. The occupational therapist is educating Jerome and his family about energy conservation techniques to use when he is discharged home. ❖

WEB RESOURCES
American Lung Association
www.lungusa.orgsite/pp.asp?c=dvLUK9O0E&b=35691

Centers for Disease Control and Prevention
www.cdc.gov/Ncidod/diseases/submenus/sub_pneumonia.htm

FURTHER READING
Lichenstein R, Suggs AH, Campbell J: Pediatric pneumonia, *Emerg Med Clin North Am* 21:437, 2003.

Shah S, Sharieff GQ: Pediatric respiratory infections, *Emerg Med Clin North Am* 25:961, 2007.

72

❖

Prader-Willi Syndrome

Epidemiology

Prader-Willi syndrome (PWS) is an uncommon genetic disorder of chromosome 15. In people with PWS the part of the brain that controls hunger does not work properly, leading to overeating. Obesity is a concern for children with PWS. Poor muscle tone and low levels of sex hormones also occur in PWS.

There is no cure for PWS, although symptoms can be minimized with diet and exercise programs, as well as growth hormones.

Impact on Performance Skills

Children with PWS may experience delays in motor skills such as the following:

- Mobility
- Strength and effort
- Energy

Children with PWS may experience delays in process skills such as the following:

- Energy
- Knowledge
- Temporal organization
- Organization of space and objects
- Adaptation

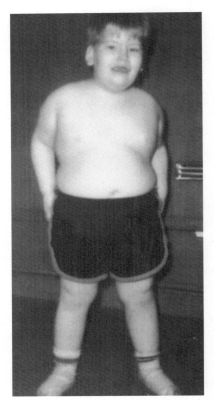

This child demonstrates the marked obesity characteristic of Prader-Willi syndrome. (From Zitelli BJ, Davis HW: *Atlas of pediatric physical diagnosis,* ed 5, St Louis, 2007, Mosby.)

Children with PWS may experience delays in communication and interaction skills such as the following:
- Physicality
- Information exchange
- Relations

P

Impact on Client Factors (Body Functions and Structures)

The part of the brain that controls feelings of fullness or hunger does not work properly in people with PWS. This results in obesity in many children with PWS.

It causes poor muscle tone, low levels of sex hormones, and a constant feeling of hunger. This can lead to obesity, which can result in heart disease and diabetes, which will limit participation.

Precautions

Impact on Performance Skills

Babies with PWS are usually floppy, with poor muscle tone, and have trouble sucking. Growth hormone and exercise can help build muscle mass and control weight. Children could have difficulty completing some activities owing to the poor muscle tone.

Impact on Client Factors (Body Functions and Structures)

Signs that may appear include the following:

- Short stature
- Poor motor skills
- Weight gain and overeating, leading to obesity
- Underdeveloped sex organs
- Mild intellectual disabilities and learning disabilities

PWS can lead a child to have difficulties with home, school, and community activities.

Evaluation

- Clinical observations
- Child-environment fit
- Child interview
- Parent or caregiver interview

Suggested Assessment Tools

- Alberta Infant Motor Scale (AIMS)
- Bayley Scale of Infant Development (BSID)
- Bruininks-Oseretsky Test of Motor Performance (BOT-2)
- Canadian Occupational Performance Measure (COPM)
- Child Occupational Self Assessment (COSA)
- Denver Developmental Screening Test (DDST)
- FirstSTEp Developmental Screening Test
- Hawaii Early Learning Profile (HELP)
- Movement Assessment Battery for Children (Movement ABC)
- Peabody Developmental Motor Scales 2, Revised (PDMS-2)
- Short Child Occupational Profile (SCOPE)
- Toddler and Infant Motor Evaluation (TIME)
- WeeFIM

INTERVENTIONS

- Environment modification and adaptation
- Task modification and adaptation
- Positioning

Case Example

Xeminia is a 2-year-old with PWS and has low tone as well as poor posture. The occupational therapist is working with Xeminia to improve her low tone and posture. ❖

WEB RESOURCES

Prader-Willi Syndrome Association
www.pwsausa.org

Center for the Study of Autism
www.autism.orgprader.html

FURTHER READING

Caliandro P, Grugni G, Padua L, et al: Quality of life assessment in a sample of patients affected by Prader-Willi syndrome, *J Paediatr Child Health* 43:826, 2007.

Lindgren AC, Barkeling B, Hägg A, et al: Eating behavior in Prader-Willi syndrome, normal weight, and obese control groups, *J Pediatr* 137:50, 2000.

Zipf WB: Prader-Willi syndrome: the care and treatment of infants, children, and adults, *Adv Pediatr* 51:409, 2004.

P

73

❖

Retinopathy of Prematurity

Epidemiology

Retinopathy of prematurity (ROP) is abnormal blood vessel development in the retina of the eye in a premature infant. The blood vessels of the retina begin to develop 3 months after conception and complete their development at the time of normal birth. When an infant is born very prematurely, the infant's eye development is disrupted.

In infants who develop ROP, the vessels grow abnormally from the retina into the normally clear gel that fills the back of the eye, which leads to fragile vessels and often hemorrhaging into the eye. This causes scar tissue, which pulls the retina loose from the inner eye and causes retinal detachment. A result of this is reduced vision or complete blindness. The condition is typically found in babies of less than 32 to 34 weeks' gestation, and a screening is typically completed on them.

Impact on Performance Skills

Children with ROP may experience delays in process skills such as the following:

- Energy
- Knowledge
- Temporal organization
- Organization of space and objects
- Adaptation

R

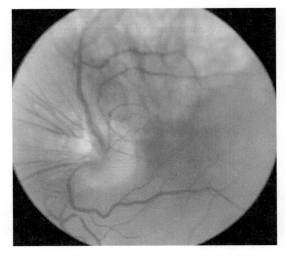

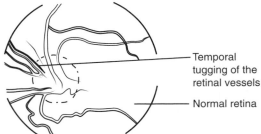

Temporal tugging of the retinal vessels

Normal retina

Retinopathy of prematurity. (From Zitelli BJ, Davis HW: *Atlas of pediatric physical diagnosis,* ed 5, St Louis, 2007, Mosby.)

Children with ROP may experience delays in communication and interaction skills such as the following:

- Physicality
- Information exchange
- Relations

Children with ROP will not have delays in process or motor skills.

Impact on Client Factors (Body Functions and Structures)

The majority of infants with mild ROP can be expected to recover completely. Severe ROP may lead to marked visual abnormalities (severe myopia [near-sightedness]) or blindness. The most important factor in the outcome is early detection and treatment.

Precautions

Impact on Performance Skills

Most children with severe vision loss from ROP have other complications of prematurity. These complications can lead to difficulties in motor, processing, and communication and interaction skills.

Impact on Client Factors (Body Functions and Structures)

Results of severe ROP may produce some of the following signs:

- White pupils
- Abnormal eye movements
- Crossed eyes

Evaluation

- Child-environment fit
- Visual screening
- Client interview
- Parent or caregiver interview
- Clinical observations

Suggested Assessment Tools

- Beery-Butenica Developmental Test of Visual-Motor Integration, Fourth Edition (VMI)
- Benton Constructional Praxis Test
- Erhardt Developmental Vision Assessment, Revised (EDVA)

R

- Motor-Free Visual Perception Test—Revised (MVPT-R)
- Test of Visual-Motor Skills: Upper Level (TVMS:UL)
- Test of Visual-Perceptual Skills (TVPS)
- Test of Visual-Perceptual Skills: Upper Level (Non-Motor) (TVPS: UL)

INTERVENTIONS

- Task modification and adaptation
- Environment modification and adaptation
- Low vision rehabilitation

Case Example

Kyle is a 3-year-old with ROP. He is having difficulty with feeding due to visual limitations. The occupational therapist is working with the family on adaptations to tasks and the home environment. ❖

WEB RESOURCES

National Eye Institute
www.nei.nih.gov/health/rop/index.asp

Association for Retinopathy of Prematurity and Related Diseases
www.ropard.org

FURTHER READING

Drack A: Retinopathy of prematurity, *Adv Pediatr* 53:211, 2006.

Rosenthal SB: Living with low vision: a personal and professional perspective, *Am J Occup Ther* 49:861, 1995.

Wheeler LC, Griffin HC, Taylor JR, Taylor S: Educational intervention strategies for children with visual impairments with emphasis on retinopathy of prematurity, *J Pediatr Health Care* 11:275, 1997.

74

❖

Rheumatic Heart Disease

Epidemiology

Rheumatic heart disease is a complication of rheumatic fever in which the heart valves are damaged. Rheumatic fever is an inflammatory disease that begins with a strep throat. It can affect connective tissue throughout the body, especially in the heart, joints, brain, and skin.

Although rheumatic fever can strike people of all ages, it is most common in children between 5 and 15 years old. The best way to prevent rheumatic fever is to treat strep throat with antibiotics.

Treatment of rheumatic heart disease may include medication and surgery. Medication will aim to avoid over-exertion. Surgery may be needed to replace the damaged valve(s).

Impact on Performance Skills

Children with rheumatic heart disease may experience delays in motor skills such as the following:

- Mobility
- Strength and effort
- Energy

Children with rheumatic heart disease may experience delays in process skills such as the following:

- Energy

Children with rheumatic heart disease will not have delays in communication and interaction skills.

Impact on Client Factors (Body Functions and Structures)

The symptoms of rheumatic heart disease vary, and damage to the heart often is not readily noticeable. When symptoms do appear, they may depend on the extent and location of the heart damage. For some children there can be fatigue and muscle weakness owing to limitations in activity. These can affect a child's motor skills.

Precautions

Impact on Performance Skills

Painful, swollen, and red joints, especially large joints, are common in children with rheumatic heart disease. Usually the symptoms go away after a couple of days, only to be replaced by the same symptoms in another joint. If the heart is affected, it is usually not severely enough to cause symptoms, although the child may be short of breath.

Impact on Client Factors (Body Functions and Structures)

Some of the most common signs and symptoms of rheumatic heart disease are as follows:
- Breathlessness
- Fatigue
- Palpitations
- Chest pain
- Fainting attacks

Rheumatic heart disease may limit a child's participation in activities within the home, school, and community.

Evaluation
- Clinical observations
- Child-environment fit

- Client interview
- Parent or caregiver interview

Suggested Assessment Tools

- Canadian Occupational Performance Measure (COPM)
- Child Behavior Checklist (CBCL)
- Child Occupational Self Assessment (COSA)
- Klein-Bell Activities of Daily Living Scale
- Pediatric Evaluation of Disability Inventory (PEDI)
- Short Child Occupational Profile (SCOPE)

INTERVENTIONS

- Task modification and adaptation
- Environment modification and adaptation
- Energy conservation

Case Example

Josh is a 7-year-old who has rheumatic heart disease. He is frequently tired and fatigued. The occupational therapist is working with Josh and his family to address his energy level and the environments he is in such as school and community activities. ❖

WEB RESOURCE

American Heart Association
www.americanheart.orgpresenter.jhtml?identifier=4709

FURTHER READING

De Rosa G, Pardeo M, Stabile A, Rigante D: Rheumatic heart disease in children: from clinical assessment to therapeutical management, *Eur Rev Med Pharmacol Sci* 10:107, 2006.

Yasumura M, Baldwin JS: Occupational therapy for rheumatic and cardiac children, *Am J Occup Ther* 7:62, 1953.

75

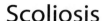

Scoliosis

Epidemiology

Scoliosis is the curvature of the spine. The spine curves away from the middle or sideways.

There are three general causes of scoliosis. Congenital scoliosis is due to a problem with the formation of vertebrae or fused ribs during prenatal development. Neuromuscular scoliosis is caused by problems such as poor muscle control or muscular weakness or paralysis due to diseases such as cerebral palsy, muscular dystrophy, spina bifida, and polio. Idiopathic scoliosis is of unknown cause and appears in a previously straight spine.

Impact on Performance Skills

Children with scoliosis may experience delays in motor skills such as the following:
- Mobility
- Strength and effort
- Energy

Children with scoliosis may experience delays in process skills such as the following:
- Energy
- Organization of space and objects

Children with scoliosis may experience delays in communication and interaction skills such as the following:

S

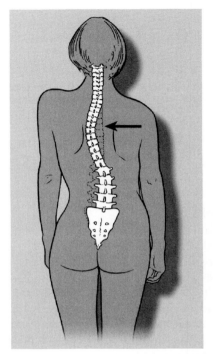

Abnormal spinal curvature: scoliosis. (From Thibodeau GA, Patton KT: *The human body in health and disease,* ed 4, St Louis, 2005, Mosby.)

- Physicality
- Relations

Impact on Client Factors (Body Functions and Structures)

Children with scoliosis may have emotional problems or lowered self-esteem. This needs to be explored in order to provide a supportive environment for children who are experiencing possible social withdrawal owing to the emotional effects of scoliosis. They also may have nerve or spinal damage from corrective surgery or even from the curvature of the spine if it goes uncorrected. At times, respiratory problems can occur from severe spinal curvatures. Fatigue and weakness can result from the respiratory problems.

Precautions

Impact on Performance Skills

Treatment depends on the cause of the scoliosis, the size and location of the curve, and how much more growing the child is expected to do. Most cases of adolescent idiopathic scoliosis (less than 20 degrees) require no treatment but should be checked often, about every 6 months.

As curves get worse (above 25 to 30 degrees in a child who is still growing), bracing is usually recommended to help slow the progression of the curve. There are many different kinds of braces used. A back brace does not reverse the curve. Instead, it uses pressure to help straighten the spine. The brace can be adjusted with growth. Bracing does not work in congenital or neuromuscular scoliosis and is less effective in infantile and juvenile idiopathic scoliosis.

Bracing can affect a child's ability to participate in activities, especially if the bracing follows a surgical procedure to straighten the spine. Adaptations to tasks and environments may be necessary.

Impact on Client Factors (Body Functions and Structures)

Prolonged sitting or standing can cause spinal fatigue. Pain will become persistent if irritation results. The greater the initial curve of the spine, the greater the chance the scoliosis will get worse after growth is complete. Severe scoliosis (curves in the spine greater than 100 degrees) may cause breathing problems.

The outcome depends on the cause, location, and severity of the curve. The greater the curve, the greater the chance the curve will get worse after growth has stopped.

Clients with mild cases treated with bracing alone do very well. People with these kinds of conditions tend not to have long-term problems, except maybe an increased rate of low back pain when they get older. People with surgically corrected idiopathic scoliosis also do very well and can lead active, healthy lives.

Children with neuromuscular scoliosis have another serious disorder (such as cerebral palsy or muscular dystrophy), so their goals are much different. Often the goal of surgery is simply to allow a child to be able to sit upright in a wheelchair.

Babies with congenital scoliosis have a wide variety of underlying birth defects. Management of this disease is difficult and often requires many surgeries.

The limitations imposed by the treatments are often emotionally difficult and may threaten self-image, especially of teenagers. Emotional support is important for adjustment to the limitations that result from scoliosis or treatment for scoliosis. Promoting participation in activities as a child is able will aid in adjusting to limitations.

Evaluation
- Clinical observations
- Child-environment fit
- Client interview

Suggested Assessment Tools
- Canadian Occupational Performance Measure (COPM)
- Klein-Bell Activities of Daily Living Scale
- Short Child Occupational Profile (SCOPE)
- WeeFIM

INTERVENTIONS
- Task modification and adaptation
- Environment modification and adaptation
- Pain management techniques
- Joint protection

Case Example

Jenny is a 14-year-old with scoliosis. She is having difficulty in school resulting from limitations in her ability to put away items during a vocational course; she also experiences extreme fatigue. The occupational therapist is working with the teacher to modify the environment to meet the needs of this student. ❖

WEB RESOURCES

National Scoliosis Foundation
www.scoliosis.org

Scoliosis World
www.scoliosis-world.com

FURTHER READING

Campos MA, Weinstein SL: Pediatric scoliosis and kyphosis, *Neurosurg Clin North Am* 18(3):515-529, 2007.

Glancy GL: Advances in idiopathic scoliosis in children and adolescents, *Adv Pediatr* 54:55-66, 2007.

Karski T, Madej J, Rehák L, et al: New conservative treatment of idiopathic scoliosis: effectiveness of therapy, *Ortop Traumatol Rehabil* 7(1):28-35, 2005.

76

❖

Separation Anxiety and Social Phobia

Epidemiology

Some measure of anxiety is a normal aspect of development. For example, most toddlers become fearful when separated from their mothers, especially in unfamiliar surroundings. Fears of the dark, monsters, bugs, and spiders are common in 3- to 4-year-olds. Shy children may initially react to new situations with fear or withdrawal. Fears of injury and death are more common in older children. Older children and adolescents often become anxious when giving a book report in front of their classmates. Such difficulties should not be viewed as evidence of a disorder.

However, when these otherwise normal manifestations of anxiety become so exaggerated that functioning becomes greatly impaired or severe distress is endured, an anxiety disorder should be considered.

Prognosis depends on severity, availability of competent treatment, and the child's resiliency. In most cases, children struggle with anxiety symptoms into adulthood and beyond. However, with early treatment many children learn how to control their anxiety.

Impact on Performance Skills

Children with separation anxiety may experience delays in communication and interaction skills such as the following:

- Physicality
- Information exchange
- Relations

Children with separation anxiety will not have delays in motor or process skills.

Impact on Client Factors (Body Functions and Structures)

Anxiety disorders seem to have a genetic basis and can be modified by psychosocial experience. Anxious parents tend to have anxious children, which has the unfortunate potential of making the child's problems worse than they otherwise might be. The focus for separation anxiety should include the parents and the child for a comprehensive approach to improving a child's ability to participate in the home, school, and community.

Precautions

Impact on Performance Skills

An upset stomach, nausea, and headaches often develop in children with anxiety. A behavior program may be necessary to help the child to address anxiety. This should be implemented under the direction of a behavior specialist.

Impact on Client Factors (Body Functions and Structures)

Children with anxiety disorders exhibit a state of fear, worry, or dread that greatly impairs functioning and is disproportionate to the circumstances at hand.

Evaluation

- Clinical observation
- Child-environment fit
- Client interview
- Parent or caregiver interview

Suggested Assessment Tools

- Classroom Observation Guide
- Nowicki-Strickland Locus of Control Scale for Children (TIM[C])
- Pediatric Volitional Questionnaire (PVQ)
- Short Child Occupational Profile (SCOPE)

INTERVENTIONS

- Environment modification and adaptation
- Behavior modification
- Family and caregiver education

Case Example

Irene is a 6-year-old who refuses to go to school, because she feels "sick." Her parents realize that Irene is not really sick but is experiencing separation anxiety. They have asked for a consultation with the school psychologist, who has asked the occupational therapist to work as part of the team to develop a plan for the child. ❖

WEB RESOURCES

Social Phobia Net
www.childanxiety.net/Social_Phobia.htm

Psychiatric Times
www.psychiatrictimes.com/showArticle.jhtml?articleID=175802533

FURTHER READING

Arnold P, Banerjee SP, Bhandari R, et al: Childhood anxiety disorders and developmental issues in anxiety, *Curr Psychiatry Rep* 5:252, 2003.

Ferdinand RF, Bongers IL, van der Ende J, et al: Distinctions between separation anxiety and social anxiety in children and adolescents, *Behav Res Ther* 44:1523, 2006.

Hanna GL, Fischer DJ, Fluent TE: Separation anxiety disorder and school refusal in children and adolescents, *Pediatr Rev* 27:56, 2006.

77

❖

Sensory Processing Disorder

Epidemiology

Sensory processing refers to our ability to take in information through our senses (touch, movement, smell, taste, vision, and hearing), organize and interpret that information, and make a meaningful response. For most people this process is automatic. Sensory processing disorder (SPD) affects the way the brain interprets the information that comes in and the response that follows, causing emotional, motor, and other reactions that are inappropriate and extreme.

Impact on Performance Skills

Children with SPD may experience delays in motor skills such as the following:

- Posture
- Mobility
- Coordination
- Strength and effort
- Energy

Children with SPD may experience delays in process skills such as the following:

- Energy
- Knowledge
- Temporal organization
- Organization of space and objects
- Adaptation

Children with SPD may experience delays in communication and interaction skills such as the following:

- Physicality
- Information exchange
- Relations

Impact on Client Factors (Body Functions and Structures)

- Oversensitivity to touch, movement, sights, or sounds
- Underreactivity to touch, movement, sights, or sounds
- Tendency to be easily distracted
- Social and/or emotional problems
- Activity level that is unusually high or unusually low
- Physical clumsiness or apparent carelessness
- Impulsivity, lack of self-control
- Difficulty in making transitions from one situation to another
- Inability to unwind or calm self
- Poor self-concept
- Delays in speech, language, or motor skills
- Delays in academic achievement

SPD makes it difficult for children to function at home, in school, or in the community because of the extreme reactions they have owing to the sensory response to information from the environment.

Precautions

Impact on Performance Skills

Children can be overresponsive or underresponsive to sensation. This leads them to feel as if they are being constantly bombarded with sensory information or that they are in need of constant sensory stimulation. Sometimes children with SPD do not notice pain or objects that are too hot or cold, and they may need high-intensity input in order to become involved in activities. Others have trouble distinguishing among different types of sensory stimulation.

Children often need to have task and environment adaptations owing to their reactions to stimuli.

Impact on Client Factors (Body Functions and Structures)

The presence of SPD is typically detected in young children. Although most affected children develop SPD during the course of ordinary childhood activities, which helps establish such things as the ability for motor planning and adapting to incoming sensations, in others such abilities do not develop as efficiently. When their process is disordered, a variety of problems in learning, development, or behavior become obvious. This can limit motor, process, and communication and interaction skills.

Evaluation

- Clinical observations
- Child-environment fit
- Parent or caregiver interview

Suggested Assessment Tools

- Adolescent/Adult Sensory Profile
- Balcones Sensory Integration Screening Kit
- DeGangi-Berk Test of Sensory Integration (TSI)
- Infant/Toddler Sensory Profile
- Short Child Occupational Profile (SCOPE)

INTERVENTIONS

- Sensory education
- Task modification and adaptation
- Environment modification and adaptation
- Family, caregiver, and child education
- Home program

Case Example _____

Sam is a 2-year-old. His mother is concerned because he cannot tolerate textures on his body, he is unable to focus on any one toy and moves aimlessly about their home. He does not engage in any purposeful activity or play. An occupational therapist has been asked to evaluate and treat Sam to improve his sensory function. ❖

WEB RESOURCES

SPD Network
www.spdnetwork.org

Sensory Processing Disorder
www.sensory-processing-disorder.com/sensory-processing-disorder-checklist.html

Sensational Kids
www.sensationalkids.org

FURTHER READING

Dunn W, Brown C: Factor analysis on the Sensory Profile from a national sample of children without disabilities, *Am J Occup Ther* 51:490, 1997.

Miller LJ, Schoen SA, James K, Schaaf RC: Lessons learned: a pilot study on occupational therapy effectiveness for children with sensory modulation disorder, *Am J Occup Ther* 61:161, 2007.

Reisman J: Sensory processing disorders, *Minn Med* 85:48, 2002.

78

❖

Sepsis

Epidemiology

Sepsis is a severe illness caused by overwhelming infection of the bloodstream by toxin-producing bacteria. Sepsis is often life-threatening, especially in children with a weakened immune system or other medical illnesses.

Impact on Performance Skills

Children with sepsis may experience delays in motor skills such as the following:
- Mobility
- Strength and effort
- Energy

Children with sepsis may experience delays in process skills such as the following:
- Energy
- Knowledge
- Temporal organization
- Organization of space and objects
- Adaptation

Children with sepsis may experience delays in communication and interaction skills such as the following:
- Physicality
- Information exchange
- Relations

Impact on Client Factors (Body Functions and Structures)

Children with sepsis usually require monitoring in an intensive care unit (ICU). Intravenous antibiotic therapy is initiated as soon as sepsis is suspected. Weakness and fatigue can cause problems with motor skills as a result of muscle atrophy.

Precautions

Impact on Performance Skills

Early warning signs of sepsis include a change in mental state and hyperventilation. Confusion, fatigue, and muscle weakness can limit a child's ability to participate in activities.

Impact on Client Factors (Body Functions and Structures)

Conditions that occur as a result of sepsis are as follows:
- Septic shock
- Impaired blood flow to vital organs (brain, heart, kidneys)
- Disseminated intravascular coagulation

Evaluation

- Clinical observations
- Child-environment fit
- Client interview
- Parent or caregiver interview

Suggested Assessment Tools

- Canadian Occupational Performance Measure (COPM)
- Child Occupational Self Assessment (COSA)
- Klein-Bell Activities of Daily Living Scale
- Short Child Occupational Profile (SCOPE)
- WeeFIM

INTERVENTIONS

- Task modification and adaptation
- Environment modification and adaptation

Case Example

Macy is a 12-year-old who was in the hospital and developed sepsis. She was placed in the pediatric intensive care unit (PICU). The occupational therapist began to work with Macy to help her regain her ability to perform basic self-care tasks. ❖

WEB RESOURCES

KidsHealth.org
**www.kidshealth.orgparent/pregnancy_newborn/medical_problems/
sepsis.html**

Surviving Sepsis
www.survivingsepsis.org

FURTHER READING

Babay HA, Twum-Danso K, Kambal AM, Al-Otaibi FE: Bloodstream infections in pediatric patients, *Saudi Med J* 26:1555, 2005.

Carlotti AP, Troster EJ, Fernandes JC, Carvalho WB: A critical appraisal of the guidelines for the management of pediatric and neonatal patients with septic shock, *Crit Care Med* 33:1182, 2005.

Maar SP: Emergency care in pediatric septic shock, *Pediatr Emerg Care* 20:617, 2004.

79

❖

Sickle Cell Anemia

Epidemiology

Sickle cell anemia is a disease in which the body produces abnormally shaped red blood cells. The cells are shaped like a crescent or sickle. Sickle cell anemia is most common in African Americans.

Impact on Performance Skills

Children with sickle cell anemia may experience delays in motor skills such as the following:

- Mobility
- Strength and effort
- Energy

Children with sickle cell anemia may experience delays in process skills such as the following:

- Energy

Children with sickle cell anemia will not experience delays in communication and interaction skills.

Impact on Client Factors (Body Functions and Structures)

Sickle cells get stuck in blood vessels, blocking blood flow. This can cause pain and organ damage. The pain can limit participation, and pain management can be used to help address any activity limitation that may occur because of the disease process.

S

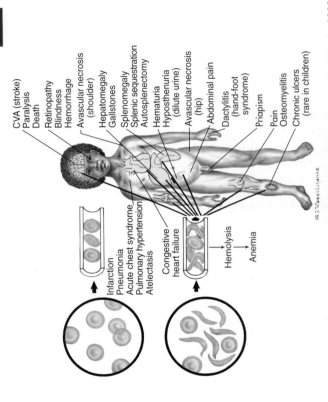

CVA (stroke)
Paralysis
Death
Retinopathy
Blindness
Hemorrhage
Avascular necrosis (shoulder)
Hepatomegaly
Gallstones
Splenomegaly
Splenic sequestration
Autosplenectomy
Hematuria
Hyposthenuria (dilute urine)
Avascular necrosis (hip)
Abdominal pain
Dactylitis (hand-foot syndrome)
Priapism
Pain
Osteomyelitis
Chronic ulcers (rare in children)

Infarction
Pneumonia
Acute chest syndrome
Pulmonary hypertension
Atelectasis
Congestive heart failure

Hemolysis → Anemia

Sickle cell anemia. (From Hockenberry MJ: *Wong's essentials of pediatric nursing*, ed 7, St Louis, 2005, Mosby.)

Precautions

Impact on Performance Skills

Sickle cells do not last as long as normal, round red blood cells, which leads to anemia. Anemia causes fatigue, which can limit participation in activities, but with task adaptation and modification participation can improve.

Impact on Client Factors (Body Functions and Structures)

See earlier section for impact on client factors.

Evaluation

- Clinical observations
- Client interview
- Parent or caregiver interview
- Child-environment fit

Suggested Assessment Tools

- Canadian Occupational Performance Measure (COPM)
- Klein-Bell Activities of Daily Living Scale
- Short Child Occupational Profile (SCOPE)
- WeeFIM

INTERVENTIONS

- Energy conservation
- Task modification and adaptation
- Environment modification and adaptation

Case Example

Lashonda is a 14-year-old with sickle cell anemia. She has been experiencing increased fatigue and pain, which are causing her to have a hard time concentrating during high school classes. The occupational therapist has been consulted and recommends that Lashonda follow an energy conservation plan throughout her day as well as exploring methods for pain management. The occupational therapist also has consulted with the school dietitian to help design an iron-rich diet that she will review with Lashonda.

WEB RESOURCES

National Heart Lung and Blood Institute
www.nhlbi.nih.gov/health/dci/Diseases/Sca/SCA_WhatIs.html

Sickle Cell Information Center
www.scinfo.org

FURTHER READING

Jacob E, Miaskowski C, Savedra M, et al: Changes in sleep, food intake and activity levels during acute painful episodes in children with sickle cell disease, *J Pediatr Nurs* 21:23, 2006.

Mitchell MJ, Lemanek K, Palermo TM, et al: Parent perspectives on pain management, coping, and family functioning in pediatric sickle cell disease, *Clin Pediatr (Phila)* 46:311, 2007.

Thompson AA: Advances in the management of sickle cell disease, *Pediatr Blood Cancer* 46:533, 2006.

Westfold F: Sickle cell disorders, *Nurs Stand* 20:67, 2006.

Yoon SL, Godwin A: Enhancing self-management in children with sickle cell disease through playing a CD-ROM educational game: a pilot study, *Pediatr Nurs* 33:60, 72, 2007.

80

❖

Spina Bifida

Epidemiology

Spina bifida is the most common disabling birth defect in the United States. It is a type of neural tube defect, which is a problem with the spinal cord or its coverings. It happens if the fetal spinal column does not close completely during the first month of pregnancy. Taking folic acid, which is in most multivitamins, can reduce the risk of having a baby with spina bifida. Women who could become pregnant should take it daily.

Impact on Performance Skills

Children with spina bifida may experience delays in motor skills such as the following:

- Posture
- Mobility
- Strength and effort
- Coordination
- Energy

Children with spina bifida may experience delays in process skills such as the following:

- Energy
- Knowledge
- Temporal organization
- Organization of space and objects
- Adaptation

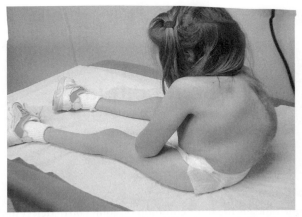

This child with thoracic-level spina bifida has an obvious kyphotic deformity. (From Zitelli BJ, Davis HW: *Atlas of pediatric physical diagnosis,* ed 5, St Louis, 2007, Mosby.)

Children with spina bifida may experience delays in communication and interaction skills such as the following:

- Physicality
- Information exchange
- Relations

Impact on Client Factors (Body Functions and Structures)

Many children with spina bifida will need assistive devices such as braces, crutches, or wheelchairs.

Precautions

Impact on Performance Skills

Spina bifida usually causes nerve damage that results in at least some paralysis of the legs. There is no cure.

Impact on Client Factors (Body Functions and Structures)

Children with spina bifida may have learning difficulties, urinary and bowel problems, or hydrocephalus, a buildup of fluid in the brain. Modifications to tasks and various environments may be necessary.

Evaluation

- Clinical observations
- Child interview
- Child-environment fit
- Parent or caregiver interview

Suggested Assessment Tools

- Alberta Infant Motor Scale (AIMS)
- Bay Area Functional Performance Evaluation (BaFPE)
- Canadian Occupational Performance Measure (COPM)
- Child Occupational Self Assessment (COSA)
- Children's Assessment of Participation and Enjoyment (CAPE)
- Classroom Observation Guide
- Denver Developmental Screening Test (DDST)
- Home Observation and Measurement of the Environment (HOME)
- Klein-Bell Activities of Daily Living Scale
- Occupational Circumstances Assessment Interview and Rating Scale (OCAIRS)
- Occupational Performance History Inventory (Version 2) (OPHI-2)
- Pediatric Evaluation of Disability Inventory (PEDI)
- Preferences for Activities of Children (PAC)
- School Function Assessment (SFA)
- School Setting Interview (SSI)
- Short Child Occupational Profile (SCOPE)
- Vineland Adaptive Behavior Scales Revised (VABS)
- WeeFIM

INTERVENTIONS

- Task modification and adaptation
- Environment modification and adaptation
- Positioning
- Joint protection
- Leisure exploration

Case Example

Michelle is a 5-year-old with spina bifida. She has been having difficulties with toileting while at kindergarten. The occupational therapist has been asked to work with her to address this concern. ❖

WEB RESOURCES

March of Dimes
www.marchofdimes.com/pnhec/4439.asp

Spina Bifida Association
**www.sbaa.orgsite/c.liKWL7PLLrF/b.2642297/k.5F7C/Spina_Bifida_
Association.htm**

FURTHER READING

Appleton PL, Minchom PE, Ellis NC, et al: The self-concept of young people with spina bifida: a population-based study, *Dev Med Child Neurol* 36:198, 1994.

Watson D: Occupational therapy intervention guidelines for children and adolescents with spina bifida, *Child Care Health Dev* 17:367, 1991.

81

❖

Spinal Muscular Atrophy

Epidemiology

Spinal muscular atrophy (SMA) is the number one genetic killer of children under the age of 2. An inherited condition, SMA is one of the most prevalent genetic disorders. SMA is classified into four types based on milestones achieved at onset of SMA. Types I and II are more prevalent.

Impact on Performance Skills

Children with SMA may experience delays in motor skills such as the following:
- Posture
- Mobility
- Strength and effort
- Coordination
- Energy

Children with SMA may experience delays in process skills such as the following:
- Energy
- Knowledge
- Temporal organization
- Organization of space and objects
- Adaptation

Children with SMA will not have delays in communication and interaction skills.

Impact on Client Factors (Body Functions and Structures)

SMA is often fatal, and it destroys the nerves controlling voluntary muscle movement. Positioning and joint protection may be needed as motor control lessens as the disease progresses.

Precautions

Impact on Performance Skills

Depending on the type of SMA, a child can have difficulties with sitting, standing or ambulating unaided, crawling, walking, controlling the head and neck, and even swallowing.

Adaptations to tasks and the environment may be necessary for children who have difficulty with sitting or standing.

Impact on Client Factors (Body Functions and Structures)

See section on Impact on Performance Skills.

Evaluation

- Parent or caregiver interview
- Child interview
- Child-environment fit

Suggested Assessment Tools

- Alberta Infant Motor Scale (AIMS)
- Bay Area Functional Performance Evaluation (BaFPE)
- Bayley Scale of Infant Development (BSID)
- Bruininks-Oseretsky Test of Motor Performance (BOT-2)
- Canadian Occupational Performance Measure (COPM)
- Child Occupational Self Assessment (COSA)
- Children's Assessment of Participation and Enjoyment (CAPE)
- Classroom Observation Guide

- Denver Developmental Screening Test (DDST)
- Early Coping Inventory
- FirstSTEp Developmental Screening Test
- Hawaii Early Learning Profile (HELP)
- Klein-Bell Activities of Daily Living Scale
- Lincoln-Oseretsky Motor Development Scale
- Miller Assessment for Preschoolers (MAP)
- Peabody Developmental Motor Scales 2, Revised (PDMS-2)
- Pediatric Evaluation of Disability Inventory (PEDI)
- Pediatric Volitional Questionnaire (PVQ)
- School Function Assessment (SFA)
- School Setting Interview (SSI)
- Short Child Occupational Profile (SCOPE)
- Toddler and Infant Motor Evaluation (TIME)
- Vineland Adaptive Behavior Scales Revised (VABS)
- WeeFIM

INTERVENTIONS

- Task modification and adaptation
- Environment modification and adaptation
- Joint protection

Case Example

Lonnie is a 4-year old with SMA. He has trouble with dressing owing to being unable to sit upright unaided. His parents would like for him to be able to do as much as he can on his own and have asked for an occupational therapist to evaluate and intervene. ❖

WEB RESOURCES

Families of Spinal Muscular Atrophy
www.fsma.org

Spinal Muscular Atrophy Foundation
www.smafoundation.org

FURTHER READING

Chung BH, Wong VC, Ip P: Spinal muscular atrophy: survival pattern and functional status, *Pediatrics* 114:e548, 2004.

Eng GD, Binder H, Koch B: Spinal muscular atrophy: experience in diagnosis and rehabilitation management of 60 patients, *Arch Phys Med Rehabil* 65:549, 1984.

Koch BM, Simenson RL: Upper extremity strength and function in children with spinal muscular atrophy type II, *Arch Phys Med Rehabil* 73:241, 1992.

S

82

❖

Strabismus

Epidemiology

Strabismus is a disorder that causes one eye to be misaligned with the other when focusing. Strabismus is caused by a lack of coordination between the eyes. As a result, the eyes look in different directions and do not focus at the same time on a single point.

In most cases of strabismus in children the cause is unknown; most often the condition is present at or shortly after birth (congenital strabismus).

Impact on Performance Skills

Children with strabismus may experience delays in process skills such as the following:

- Energy
- Knowledge
- Temporal organization
- Organization of space and objects
- Adaptation

Children with strabismus may experience delays in communication and interaction skills such as the following:

- Physicality
- Information exchange
- Relations

Children with strabismus will not have delays in motor skills.

Impact on Client Factors (Body Functions and Structures)

- Eyes that appear crossed
- Eyes that do not align in the same direction
- Uncoordinated eye movements
- Double vision
- Vision in only one eye, with loss of depth perception

Precautions

Impact on Performance Skills

In children, when the two eyes fail to focus on the same image, the brain may learn to ignore the input from one eye. If this is allowed to continue, the eye that the brain ignores will never see well.

Impact on Client Factors (Body Functions and Structures)

There may be embarrassment over facial appearance because the child will need to wear an eye patch to help correct the problem. An early diagnosis and intervention can correct the defect. With delayed treatment, vision loss in one eye may be permanent.

Evaluation

- Visual skills
- Child interview
- Parent or caregiver interview
- Child-environment fit

Suggested Assessment Tools

- Beery-Butenica Developmental Test of Visual-Motor Integration, Fourth Edition (VMI)
- Developmental Test of Visual Perception, Second Edition (DTVP-2)
- Erhardt Developmental Vision Assessment, Revised (EDVA)

- Motor-Free Visual Perception Test—Revised (MVPT-R)
- Test of Visual-Perceptual Skills (Non-Motor) (TVPS)

INTERVENTIONS

- Visual rehabilitation
- Task modification and adaptation
- Environment modification and adaptation
- Leisure exploration

Case Example

Garrett is a 7-year-old with strabismus. His parents did not seek services for this issue before he entered school. The occupational therapist is to evaluate Garrett and intervene as needed to improve his participation in school and the community and his self-care. ❖

WEB RESOURCES

Optometrists Network
www.strabismus.org

EyeMDLink.com
www.eyemdlink.com/Condition.asp?ConditionID=421

American Association for Pediatric Ophthalmology and Strabismus
www.aapos.org

FURTHER READING

Kushner BJ: Perspective on strabismus, 2006, *Arch Ophthalmol* 124:1321, 2006.

Titomanlio L, Evrard P, Mercier JC: Pediatric strabismus, *N Engl J Med* 356:2750, 2007.

83

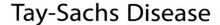

Tay-Sachs Disease

Epidemiology

Tay-Sachs disease is a fatal disease passed down through families, causing damage to the nervous system. The disease occurs when the body lacks hexosaminidase A, a protein that helps break down a chemical found in nerve tissue called *gangliosides*. Without this protein, gangliosides, particularly ganglioside GM2, build up in cells, especially nerve cells in the brain.

Tay-Sachs disease is due to a defective gene on chromosome 15. When both parents carry the defective Tay-Sachs gene, a child has a 25% chance of developing the disease. The child must receive two copies of the defective gene in order to become sick. If only one parent passes the defective gene to the child, the child is called a *carrier*. Anyone can be a carrier of Tay-Sachs. However, the rate of the disease is much higher among the Ashkenazi Jewish population.

There is no treatment for Tay-Sachs disease itself; there are only ways to make the patient more comfortable. Children affected with this disease have progressive symptoms and usually die by 4 or 5 years of age.

Impact on Performance Skills

Children with Tay-Sachs disease may experience delays in motor skills such as the following:

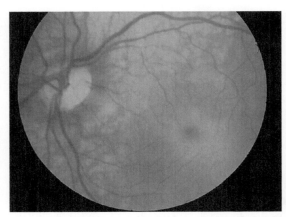

Tay-Sachs disease produces a cherry-red spot in the macula. (From Zitelli BJ, Davis HW: *Atlas of pediatric physical diagnosis,* ed 5, St Louis, 2007, Mosby.)

- Posture
- Mobility
- Strength and effort
- Coordination
- Energy

Children with Tay-Sachs disease may experience delays in process skills such as the following:

- Energy
- Knowledge
- Temporal organization
- Organization of space and objects
- Adaptation

Children with Tay-Sachs disease may experience delays in communication and interaction skills such as the following:

- Physicality
- Information exchange
- Relations

Impact on Client Factors (Body Functions and Structures)

Most people with Tay-Sachs have the infantile form. In this form the nerve damage usually begins while the fetus is still in the womb. Signs usually appear when the child is 3 to 6 months old. The disease tends to get worse very quickly, and the child usually dies by age 4 or 5. Adaptation to the environment and tasks can be provided as well as family support as the disease progresses.

T

Precautions

Impact on Performance Skills

As the disease progresses, children will exhibit spasticity and seizures as well as loss of all voluntary movement. The focus should be comfort measures for the child in the form of positioning and joint protection.

Impact on Client Factors (Body Functions and Structures)

See section on Impact on Performance Skills.

Evaluation
- Clinical observations
- Parent or caregiver interview
- Child-environment fit

Suggested Assessment Tools
- Alberta Infant Motor Scale (AIMS)
- Bayley Scale of Infant Development (BSID)
- Canadian Occupational Performance Measure (COPM)
- Denver Developmental Screening Test (DDST)
- Hawaii Early Learning Profile (HELP)
- Klein-Bell Activities of Daily Living Scale

- Lincoln-Oseretsky Motor Development Scale
- Movement Assessment for Infants (MAI)
- Peabody Developmental Motor Scales 2, Revised (PDMS-2)
- Pediatric Evaluation of Disability Inventory (PEDI)
- Short Child Occupational Profile (SCOPE)
- Toddler and Infant Motor Evaluation (TIME)
- Vineland Adaptive Behavior Scales Revised (VABS)
- WeeFIM

INTERVENTIONS

- Task modification and adaptation
- Environment modification and adaptation
- Joint protection
- Positioning

Case Example

Daniel is 7 months old. He has been diagnosed with Tay-Sachs. The occupational therapist has made recommendations to the family concerning positioning and joint protection due to Daniel's limited movement. ❖

WEB RESOURCES

National Tay-Sachs and Allied Diseases Association
www.ntsad.org

Genetics Home Reference

March of Dimes
www.marchofdimes.com/pnhec/4439_1227.asp

FURTHER READING

Aronsont SM: Early epidemiologic studies of Tay-Sachs disease, *Adv Genet* 44:25, 2001.

Fernandes Filho JA, Shapiro BE: Tay-Sachs disease, *Arch Neurol* 61:1466, 2004.

Kaback MM, Desnick RJ: Tay-Sachs disease: from clinical description to molecular defect, *Adv Genet* 44:1, 2001.

Weinstein LB: Selected genetic disorders affecting Ashkenazi Jewish families, *Fam Community Health* 30:50, 2007.

T

84

Tourette Syndrome

Epidemiology

Tourette syndrome causes children to make unusual movements or sounds, called *tics*. About one of every 100 people has Tourette syndrome. The cause of Tourette syndrome is unknown, but it is more common in boys than in girls. The tics usually start in childhood and may be worst in the early teens. Many children eventually outgrow them.

Impact on Performance Skills

Children with Tourette syndrome may experience delays in communication and interaction skills such as the following:

- Physicality
- Information exchange
- Relations

Children with Tourette syndrome will not have delays in motor skills and process skills.

Impact on Client Factors (Body Functions and Structures)

Excitement or worry can make tics worse. Calm, focused activities and structure can help improve a child's participation.

Precautions

Impact on Performance Skills

Children have little or no control over tics. Adaptation to the environment may be necessary to enhance skills.

Impact on Client Factors (Body Functions and Structures)

Common tics are throat-clearing and blinking, repeating words, spinning, or, rarely, blurting swear words.

Evaluation

- Client interview
- Child-environment fit

Suggested Assessment Tools

- Canadian Occupational Performance Measure (COPM)
- Klein-Bell Activities of Daily Living Scale
- Short Child Occupational Profile (SCOPE)
- WeeFIM

INTERVENTIONS

- Environment modification and adaptation
- Task modification and adaptation

No treatment is needed unless the tics interfere with everyday life.

Case Example

Eric is 8 years old and has Tourette syndrome. At times he yells out in class and exhibits physical tics. The occupational therapist consults with the classroom teacher to provide the best environmental fit for Eric to participate fully in the learning process. ❖

WEB RESOURCES

Tourette Syndrome Association
www.tsa-usa.org

Tourette-syndrome.com
www.tourette-syndrome.com

FURTHER READING

Rampello L, Alvano A, Battaglia G, et al: Tic disorders: from pathophysiology to treatment, *J Neurol* 253(1):1-15, 2006.

Robertson MM: Tourette syndrome, associated conditions and the complexities of treatment, *Brain* 123(Pt 3):425, 2000.

Shavitt RG, Hounie AG, Rosário Campos MC, Miguel EC: Tourette's syndrome, *Psychiatr Clin North Am,* 29:471, 2006.

Swain JE, Scahill L, Lombroso PJ, et al: Tourette syndrome and tic disorders: a decade of progress, *J Am Acad Child Adolesc Psychiatry* 46:947, 2007.

T

Appendices

A

❖

Websites for Research

American Occupational Therapy Association
www.aota.org
The AOTA website contains information that represents the interests of occupational therapy practitioners and students of occupational therapy. There is general information for practitioners, educators, researchers, students, and consumers about the occupational therapy field.

American Occupational Therapy Foundation
www.aotf.org
The AOTF is a nonprofit organization devoted to the promotion of scientific advances in occupational therapy and increasing public understanding of the field. The AOTF website houses news about occupational therapy for students and practitioners as well as updates about and achievements in research supported by the foundation.

CanChild Centre for Disability Research
www.canchild.ca
CanChild is a transdisciplinary organization devoted to youth with physical, developmental, and communication needs and their families. CanChild seeks to conduct and provide leadership in research to improve the lives of children with disabilities. The CanChild website offers important information about research supported by the foundation and its donors.

Centers for Disease Control and Prevention
www.cdc.gov
Government-run online resource for transdisciplinary health information. The site examines and defines diseases and health issues, including many of those discussed in this handbook.

Cochrane Reviews
www.cochrane.org
Cochrane Reviews is an international nonprofit independent organization dedicated to providing current and accurate information about the effects of interventions and making this information readily available to practitioners and consumers. This site provides comprehensive reviews of health care interventions and promotes the pursuit of evidence through clinical trials and other methods of investigation.

Google Scholar
http://scholar.google.com
A freely accessible search engine that indexes the full text of free transdisciplinary scholarly literature provided in an array of publishing formats.

Model of Human Occupation Clearinghouse
www.moho.uic.edu
MOHO Clearinghouse is a nonprofit organization that provides students, practitioners, educators, and researchers with information and resources related to the Model of Human Occupation.

National Institute of Health: PubMed Central
www.pubmedcentral.nih.gov
A free digital archive of biomedical and life sciences journal literature at the U.S. National Institutes of Health (NIH), developed and managed by NIH's National Center for Biotechnology Information (NCBI) in the National Library of Medicine (NLM).

OT Critically Appraised Topics
www.otcats.com
This site contains critically appraised topics and critically appraised papers focusing on occupational therapy interventions. Topics and papers are based on the best available research evidence and usually include more than one study.

OT Seeker
www.otseeker.com
A free database that provides abstracts related to a specific clinical question or keyword search. OT Seeker provides appraisals for each study and a rating to help therapists interpret the validity of the findings. OT Seeker also provides an expansive list of other websites.

U.S. Library of National Medicine
http://medlineplus.gov
MedlinePlus provides information to help answer health questions by bringing together authoritative information from the National Library of Medicine, the National Institutes of Health, and other government agencies, as well as other health-related organizations. MedlinePlus gives easy access to medical journal articles as well as extensive information about drugs, an illustrated medical encyclopedia, interactive patient tutorials, and latest health news.

Wrightslaw Special Education Law and Advocacy
www.wrightslaw.com
Wrightslaw has information about special education law, education law, and advocacy for children with disabilities. Houses thousands of articles, cases, and resources about dozens of topics relevant to school practice.

B

❖

Assessment Tools

Adolescent Role Assessment (ARA)

A test that gathers information on the adolescent's occupational role involvement over time and across domains. It is useful in screening adolescents to identify those who may be at high risk. The occupational choice process is discussed.

Alberta Infant Motor Scale (AIMS)

The Alberta Infant Motor Scale (AIMS) is an observational assessment scale constructed to measure gross motor maturation in infants from birth through independent walking.

Árnadóttir OT-ADL Neurobehavioral Evaluation (A-ONE)

The A-ONE identifies neurobehavioral deficits, the effect they have on functional performance of activities of daily living (ADLs), and how they relate to the location of cortical lesions.

Assessment of Communication and Interaction Skills (ACIS)

The ACIS is an observational assessment method that gathers data on communication and interaction skills spanning across three domains: physicality, information exchange, and relations. Each of the domains is used to describe different aspects of communication and interaction. The ACIS gathers data on skills that are exhibited during performance in an occupational form and/or within a social group.

Assessment of Ludic Behaviors (ALB)

The ALB assesses play behaviors of children with disabilities.

Assessment of Motor and Process Skills (AMPS)

The AMPS is an observational assessment used to measure the quality of performance of a person's activities of daily living by rating effort, efficiency, safety, and independence.

Balcones Sensory Integration Screening Kit

The Balcones Sensory Integration Screening Kit assists with the identification of children who might benefit from sensory-motor or sensory integrative testing and intervention. The test is appropriate for children in kindergarten through twelfth grade. There are eight major component categories, including gross motor, fine motor, and perceptual motor items.

Bay Area Functional Performance Evaluation (BaFPE)

The BaFPE is an assessment designed to evaluate the functional performance of adolescents and adults with neurologic or psychosocial impairments.

Bayley Scale of Infant Development (BSID)

The BSID assesses cognitive and motor development of infants up to 42 months old. Test items are organized in three domains: cognitive, motor, and behavioral.

Beery-Butenica Developmental Test of Visual-Motor Integration (VMI)

The VMI is used to assess visual-motor integration deficits. In practice it is used by occupational therapists, as well as psychologists, learning disability specialists, school counselors, and teachers.

Behavior Assessment Rating Scale (BASC)

The BASC is the rating scale used to identify behavior problem in children and youth, including those related to attention deficit hyperactivity disorder.

Behavioral Assessment of the Dysexecutive Syndrome (BADS)

The BADS is intended for use by occupational therapists, speech-language pathologists, and psychologists and was designed as a battery that overcomes deficiencies associated with other similar tests. The BADS includes items that are specifically sensitive to executive functions typically involved in everyday activities, such as problem solving, planning, and organizing behavior, over an extended period of time.

Benton Constructional Praxis Test

The Benton Constructional Praxis Test assesses three-dimensional visual motor and constructional skills.

Box and Block Test

The Box and Block Test assesses manual dexterity. The test provides a baseline for upper extremity manual dexterity and upper extremity gross motor coordination.

Bruininks-Oseretsky Test of Motor Performance (BOT-2)

The BOT-2 is used by occupational and physical therapists in clinics and school-based settings. The BOT-2 assesses fine and gross motor skills of children and youth (4 through 21 years of age). It is intended for use by practitioners and researchers to evaluate and characterize motor performance, specifically in the areas of fine manual control, manual coordination, body coordination, and strength and agility.

Canadian Occupational Performance Measure (COPM)

The COPM is an individualized, client-centered measure designed for use by occupational therapists to detect changes in a client's self-perception of occupational performance over time. It is designed to be used as an outcome measure and with clients with a variety of disabilities and across all developmental stages.

Child and Adolescent Social Perception Measure

The CASP was developed to provide a clinically useful measure that examines social perception within a seminaturalistic context.

Child Behavior Checklist (CBCL)

The CBCL is a standardized caregiver report that is used to identify and define problem behavior in children.

Child Behaviors Inventory of Playfulness (CBI)

The CBI is a questionnaire that is used to assess traits related to playfulness.

Child Occupational Self Assessment (COSA)

The COSA self-rating system is designed to document a child's everyday occupational participation and competence using familiar visual symbols and child-friendly language. The COSA is used in clinics and school-based settings and can be helpful in developing client-centered goals and intervention plans.

Children's Assessment of Participation and Enjoyment (CAPE)

The CAPE is the companion assessment to the Preferences for Activities of Children (PAC). The CAPE is a self-report measure of children's participation in recreation and leisure activities outside of the typical school day.

Children's Handwriting Evaluation Scale (CHES)

The CHES is used by occupational therapists and other education professionals to identify handwriting problems in children in primary grades.

Children's Paced Auditory Serial Addition Test (CHIPASAT)

The CHIPASAT is used to detect subtle impairments in attention and processing speed during observations of everyday activities.

Choosing Outcomes and Accommodations for Children (COACH)

COACH is a planning tool that is focused on meaningful outcomes such as social relationships and participation in typical home, school, and community activities. The COACH can assist in developing an individualized education plan (IEP).

Classroom Observation Guide

The Classroom Observation Guide evaluates the various interpersonal interactions among educators, interpersonal interactions among students, and interpersonal interactions between students and educators.

Computer System Usability Questionnaire

The Computer System Usability Questionnaire is used to evaluate user satisfaction with a computer program.

Coping Inventory

The Coping Inventory assesses behavior patterns and skills used by children ages 3 to 16 to meet personal needs and adapt to their environments. It measures three coping styles, including productive/nonproductive, active/passive, and flexible/rigid.

DeGangi-Berk Test of Sensory Integration (TSI)

The DeGangi-Berk Test of Sensory Integration is used for early detection of sensory processing deficits that could lead to later learning difficulties. The test is appropriate for children ages 3 to 5.

Denver Developmental Screening Test (DDST)

The DDST assesses the developmental progress of children 0 to 6 years of age.

Developmental Test of Visual Perception (DTVP)

The Developmental Test of Visual Perception measures visual perception and motor integration skills.

Dynamic Occupational Therapy Cognitive Assessment for Children (DOTCA-Ch)

The DOTCA-Ch consists of 22 subtests in five cognitive areas: orientation, spatial perception, praxis, visual motor organization, and thinking operations.

Early Coping Inventory

The Early Coping Inventory focuses on coping patterns and coping competencies for children ages 4 to 36 months. The scale rates sensorimotor organization, reactive behaviors, and self-initiated behaviors.

Erhardt Developmental Prehension Assessment (EDPA)

The EDPA measures components of arm and hand development in children of all ages and is appropriate for use with children of all cognitive and developmental levels.

Erhardt Developmental Vision Assessment, Revised (EDVA)

The EDVA measures the components of visual development in children of all ages and is appropriate for use with children of all cognitive and developmental levels.

Evaluation Tool of Children's Handwriting (ETCH)

The Evaluation Tool of Children's Handwriting evaluates six different areas of children's handwriting.

Experience of Leisure Scale (TELS)

The TELS is used by occupational therapists to assess the leisure experiences of adolescents. The TELS can also be used with adults.

Fine Motor Task Assessment

The Fine Motor Task Assessment is appropriate for use with school-aged children and provides occupational therapists with a clinical picture of a child's fine motor development.

FirstSTEp Developmental Screening Test

The FirstSTEp Developmental Screening Test identifies pre-schoolers at risk for developmental delays.

Functional Independence Measure (WeeFIM)

The WeeFIM was developed to assess functional independence in children aged 6 months to 7 years. The WeeFIM can be administered through direct observation or interview.

Gross Motor Function Measure (GMFM)

The GMFM is a clinical measure designed to assess changes in gross motor function in children with cerebral palsy.

Hawaii Early Learning Profile (HELP)

The HELP is a curriculum-based assessment of cognitive skills, language skills, gross motor skills, fine motor skills, social skills, and self-help skills for children from birth to 6 years old.

Home Observation and Measurement of the Environment (HOME)

The HOME is a semistructured caregiver interview in which the parents are asked about daily routines and other activities to assess the effect of the home environment in relation to the child's needs.

Infant/Toddler Sensory Profile

The Infant/Toddler Sensory Profile is a caregiver questionnaire that measures the sensory responses of children from infancy to 6 months of age in everyday life.

Interest Checklist

Interest Checklists are used to gauge the level of a child's interest in various topics and with various activities.

Klein-Bell Activities of Daily Living Scale

The Klein-Bell Activities of Daily Living Scale is a test used to assess independent functioning.

Knox Cube Test

The Knox Cube Test measures nonverbal, short-term memory and attention.

Knox Preschool Play Scale

The Knox Preschool Play Scale is an observational assessment administered in a naturalistic setting. The scale assesses children from birth to 6 years old and provides a developmental reference for play skills.

Leisure Boredom Scale (LBS)

The Leisure Boredom Scale contains questions about perceptions of leisure and use of leisure time.

Leisure Competence Measure

The Leisure Competence Measure was designed to measure client leisure functioning across a variety of domains.

Leisure Diagnostic Battery

The Leisure Diagnostic Battery is a leisure assessment instrument.

Leisure Satisfaction Scale

The Leisure Satisfaction Scale is an instrument used to identify leisure activities a client enjoys.

Lincoln-Oseretsky Motor Development Scale

The Lincoln-Oseretsky Motor Development Scale is an individually administered test that assesses the development of motor skills in children and adults. Areas covered include fine and gross motor skills, finger dexterity and speed, and hand-eye coordination. The test consists of 36 tasks arranged in order of increasing difficulty.

Lowenstein Occupational Therapy Cognitive Assessment (LOTCA)

The LOTCA is a test battery that is used with children ages 6 years and up. It is used to identify a child's cognitive processing.

Mayo-Portland Adaptability Inventory (MPAI)

The MPAI was designed to assist in the clinical evaluation of people during the posthospital period after a brain injury and to assist in the development of a treatment program.

McCarthy Scale of Children's Abilities

The McCarthy Scale of Children's Abilities was designed to assess the abilities of preschool children. The results of the MSCA produce six scale scores: verbal, perceptual-performance, quantitative, general cognitive, memory, and motor skills.

Miller Assessment for Preschoolers (MAP)

The MAP is a comprehensive test battery that assesses preschoolers for mild to moderate developmental delays. Basic motor skills, oral motor abilities, memory and comprehension, and sensorimotor development are evaluated through this test.

Miller Function and Participation Scales (M-FUN-S)

The M-FUN-S assesses a child's functional performance in relation to school participation in a naturalistic setting. The test links performance of functional motor activities to neuromotor foundational abilities and can be used to monitor progress over time.

Model of Human Occupation Screening Tool (MOHOST)

The MOHOST is an observational tool and was developed to be used in acute care settings. The MOHOST seeks to evaluate a client's occupational progress and assists clinicians in treatment and discharge planning.

Mother-Child Interaction Checklist

The Mother-Child Interaction Checklist provides occupational therapists with a structured format to observe interactions between a child and his or her primary caregiver.

Motor Assessment Battery for Children (Movement ABC)

The Movement ABC is used with children from 4 to 12 years old to identify movement problems that can influence a child's participation and social adjustment at school.

Movement Assessment for Infants (MAI)

The MAI is an early detection test of neurologic disorders for infants with extremely low birth weight.

NIH Activity Record

The NIH Activity Record was developed to use with people who have a physical disability and asks questions pertaining to pain, fatigue, and difficulty of daily living. The Record provides information about how a disability influences the daily activities of a client.

Nowicki-Strickland Locus of Control Scale for Children (TIM[C])

The TIM(C) is used by occupational therapists to better understand the factors that children ages 3 through 21 feel they control in daily life situations.

Occupational Circumstances Assessment Interview and Rating Scale (OCAIRS)

The OCAIRS provides a structure for gathering, analyzing, and reporting data on an individual's occupational adaptation and can be used to assess a wide age range of clients from adolescence to adulthood.

Occupational Performance History Interview (OPHI)

The OPHI was designed to gather an accurate, clinically useful history of an individual's work, play, and self-care performance. It can be used with adolescents who have disabilities.

Peabody Developmental Motor Scales 2 (PDMS-2)

The PDMS-2 is a tool used with children from birth to 5 years of age to assess gross and fine motor skills.

Pediatric Activity Card Sort (PACS)

The PACS is a pediatric self-report assessment that enables the therapist to focus intervention at the occupational level by focusing on the child's interests.

Pediatric Evaluation of Disability Inventory (PEDI)

The PEDI was developed to provide a comprehensive clinical assessment of key functional capabilities and performance in children between the ages of 6 months and 7 years. It can also be used for the evaluation of older children with significant functional limitations. The PEDI measures both capability and performance of functional activities in three domains: self-care, mobility, and social function.

Pediatric Interest Profile (PIP)

Occupational therapists use the PIP with children ages 6 to 21 to gain a better understanding of their interests.

Pediatric Volitional Questionnaire (PVQ)

The PVQ is an observation-based assessment that examines the influence of the environment on a child's volitional behavior. It can be used with all children but is particularly useful for children who, owing to age or disability, have limited communication abilities.

Perceived Efficacy and Goal Setting System (PEGS)

The PEGS involves children 6 to 9 years of age and their families in identifying priorities for intervention. The test enables the child, parent, and teacher to participate in reporting performance and identifying goals for intervention. The tool can be used with children who experience a wide range of disabilities and provides young children with disabilities the opportunity to share their perceptions of their current performance level on daily activities.

Preferences for Activities for Children (PACS)

The PACS is the companion assessment to the CAPE test. The PACS differs in that it taps into children's preferences for involvement in each activity.

Preschool and Kindergarten Behavior Scales (PKBS)

The PKBS ratings scales are designed to measure both problem behaviors and social skills of children ages 3 to 6 years of age.

School Assessment of Motor and Process Skills (School AMPS)

The School AMPS is a valid, reliable, and clinically useful tool for measuring student's schoolwork and task performance in the classroom setting. The School AMPS is a naturalistic, observation-based assessment conducted in the context of a student's regular classroom, during his or her typical routine, while the student performs schoolwork and tasks as assigned by the teacher.

School Function Assessment (SFA)

The SFA is designed to identify strengths and needs of elementary students with disabilities by examining their participation in important educationally related tasks.

School Sensory Profile

The School Sensory Profile provides a standard method for occupational therapists to measure a child's (from 5 to 10 years of age) sensory processing abilities and to explain the effect of sensory processing during daily life activities.

School Setting Interview (SSI)

The SSI is an occupational therapy assessment developed to examine the level of student-environment fit and is used in school settings. The SSI was developed for students from 10 years of age and up with physical disabilities who have some type of motor dysfunction.

Self-Assessment of Occupational Functioning (SAOF)

The Self-Assessment of Occupational Functioning is a 23-item self-assessment geared at providing insights into a child's or adolescent's own perceptions of strengths and weaknesses relative to occupational functioning.

Sensory Processing Measure (SPM)

The SPM is a standardized assessment that assists educational personnel in examining the sensory and environmental issues that may be influencing a child's performance at school and in the home.

Sensory Profile

The Sensory Profile is a caregiver questionnaire that measures children's responses to sensory events in everyday life and is appropriate for children 3 to 10 years of age.

Short Child Occupational Profile (SCOPE)

The SCOPE is a rating scale that helps an occupational therapist identify a child's strengths and occupational difficulties. It can also be used to document changes in occupational participation over time.

Social Skills Rating System

The Social Skills Rating System is an instrument developed to provide a comprehensive picture of disabled students and their social behaviors in reference to typically developing students. This rating scale allows educators to rate the occurrence and importance of specific social skills, problem behaviors, and academic competence.

Test of Environmental Supportiveness

The Test of Environmental Supportiveness is used to compare playfulness and the environment's support of play in children with and without developmental disabilities.

Test of Everyday Attention for Children (TEA-Ch)

TEA-Ch is a gamelike test used to assess different types of attention in children and adolescents aged 6 to 16 who have been diagnosed with or are suspected to have attention difficulties.

Test of Visual-Motor Skills: Upper Level (TVMS:UL)

The TVMS:UL is a copying tool used to assess clients from 12 to 40 years of age for visual motor coordination deficits that may be a result of poor motor control, delayed or impaired motor coordination, poor motor accuracy, and/or motor confusion.

Test of Visual-Perceptual Skills (TVPS-3)

The TVPS-3 is used to determine a child's visual perceptual strengths and weaknesses.

Test of Visual-Perceptual Skills: Upper Level (Nonmotor) (TVPS:UL)

The TVPS:UL is a nonmotor test used to assess clients from 12 to 40 years of age for visual perceptual deficits that may be a result of poor visual discrimination, visual memory, visual-spatial relations, visual form constancy, visual sequential memory, visual figure ground, and/or visual closure.

Toddler and Infant Motor Evaluation (TIME)

TIME is an assessment used to measure changes in children from birth to $3\frac{1}{2}$ years old who have atypical motor development. The test evaluates the relationship of motor ability to functional performance.

Vineland Adaptive Behavior Scale (VABS)

The VABS was designed to assess communication, socialization, motor skills, and performance in activities of daily living for individuals (birth through adulthood) with disabilities.

Index

A

AAI (atlantoaxial instability), in Down syndrome, 147
ABI. *See* Acquired brain injury (ABI).
Abnormal heart rates. *See* Dysrhythmias.
Abscesses, lung, due to pneumonia, 304
Achondroplasia,
    assessment tools for, 18
    body functions and structures affected by, 17, 18
    case example of, 19b
    epidemiology of, 17
    etiology of, 15
    evaluation of, 18
    interventions for, 19b
    performance skills affected by, 17, 18
    precautions with, 18
    web resources on, 19
ACIS (Assessment of Communication and Interaction Skills), 371
Acquired brain injury (ABI),
    assessment tools for, 22
    body functions and structures affected by, 22
    case example of, 24b
    epidemiology of, 21
    etiology of, 21
    evaluation of, 22
    interventions for, 23b
    performance skills affected by, 21
    precautions with, 22
    web resources on, 24
Acquired immunodeficiency syndrome (AIDS),
    assessment tools for, 26
    body functions and structures affected by, 25
    case example of, 27b
    epidemiology of, 25
    etiology of, 21

Acquired immunodeficiency syndrome (AIDS) *(Continued)*
    evaluation of, 26
    interventions for, 27b
    medical treatment of, 21
    performance skills affected by, 25
    precautions with, 26
    web resources on, 27
ADHD. *See* Attention deficit/hyperactivity disorder (ADHD).
Adolescent Role Assessment (ARA), 371
AIDS. *See* Acquired immunodeficiency syndrome (AIDS).
AIMS (Alberta Infant Motor Scale), 371
ALB (Assessment of Ludic Behaviors), 372
Albers-Schönberg disease,
    assessment tools for, 30
    body functions and structures affected by, 30
    case example of, 31b
    clinical features of, 29
    diagnosis of, 29
    epidemiology of, 29
    evaluation of, 30
    infantile, 29
    intermediate, 29
    interventions for, 31b
    medical treatment of, 29
    performance skills affected by, 29
    precautions with, 30
    web resources on, 31
Alberta Infant Motor Scale (AIMS), 371
Alcohol-related birth defects (ARBD), 161
Alcohol-related neurodevelopmental disorder (ARND), 161
Amblyopia,
    assessment tools for, 34
    body functions and structures affected by, 34

Page numbers followed by *f, t,* and *b* indicate figures, tables, and boxed material, respectively.

Amblyopia *(Continued)*
case example of, 35b
clinical features of, 33
epidemiology of, 33
etiology of, 33
evaluation of, 34
interventions for, 34b
medical treatment of, 33
performance skills affected by, 33
precautions with, 34
web resources on, 35
American Occupational Therapy
Association (AOTA) website,
367
American Occupational Therapy
Foundation (AOTF) website,
367
AMPS (Assessment of Motor and
Process Skills), 372
Anemia,
assessment tools for, 38
body functions and structures
affected by, 38
case example of, 39b
epidemiology of, 37
etiology of, 37
evaluation of, 38
interventions for, 38b
performance skills affected by, 37
precautions with, 38
sickle cell (*See* Sickle cell anemia)
web resources on, 39
Angelman syndrome,
assessment tools for, 42
body functions and structures
affected by, 42
case example of, 44b
clinical features of, 41, 43f
epidemiology of, 41
etiology of, 41
evaluation of, 42
interventions for, 44b
performance skills affected by, 41
precautions with, 42
web resources on, 44
Anorexia,
areas of occupation affected by, 45
assessment tools for, 47
body functions and structures
affected by, 46
case example of, 47b
clinical features of, 45
epidemiology of, 45
etiology of, 45
evaluation of, 46

Anorexia *(Continued)*
interventions for, 47b
performance skills affected by, 45
precautions with, 46
web resource on, 47
Anxiety,
assessment tools for, 50
body functions and structures
affected by, 50
case example of, 51b
clinical features of, 49
defined, 49
epidemiology of, 49
etiology of, 49
evaluation of, 50
interventions for, 51b
performance skills affected by, 49
precautions with, 50
web resources on, 51
Anxiety disorders,
assessment tools for, 329
body functions and structures
affected by, 328
case example of, 329b
epidemiology of, 327
evaluation of, 328
interventions for, 329b
performance skills affected by, 327,
328
precautions with, 328
web resources on, 329
A-ONE (Árnadóttir OT-ADL
Neurobehavioral Evaluation),
371
Aorta, coarctation of, 119
Aortic stenosis, 119
AOTA (American Occupational
Therapy Association) website,
367
AOTF (American Occupational
Therapy Foundation) website,
367
Apnea,
assessment tools for, 54
body functions and structures
affected by, 54
case example of, 55b
central, 53
defined, 53
epidemiology of, 53
evaluation of, 54
interventions for, 55b
mixed, 53
obstructive, 53
performance skills affected by, 54

Apnea *(Continued)*
  precautions with, 54
  web resources on, 55
ARA (Adolescent Role Assessment),
    371
ARBD (alcohol-related birth defects),
    161
Árnadóttir OT-ADL Neurobehavioral
    Evaluation (A-ONE), 371
ARND (alcohol-related
    neurodevelopmental disorder),
    161
Arrhythmias. *See* Dysrhythmias.
Arthritis, juvenile rheumatoid. *See*
    Juvenile rheumatoid arthritis
    (JRA).
Arthrogryposis multiplex congenita,
  areas of occupation affected by, 57
  assessment tools for, 59
  body functions and structures
    affected by, 59
  case example of, 60b
  clinical features of, 57, 58f
  epidemiology of, 57
  etiology of, 57
  evaluation of, 59
  interventions for, 60b
  performance skills affected by, 58
  precautions with, 59
  web resources on, 60
ASDs. *See* Autism spectrum disorder(s)
    (ASDs).
Asperger's syndrome, 74
Assessment of Communication
    and Interaction Skills (ACIS),
    371
Assessment of Ludic Behaviors (ALB),
    372
Assessment of Motor and Process Skills
    (AMPS), 372
Asthma,
  assessment tools for, 64
  body functions and structures
    affected by, 64
  case example of, 65b
  clinical features of, 63
  epidemiology of, 63
  evaluation of, 64
  interventions for, 64b
  performance patterns affected by,
    63
  performance skills affected by, 63
  precautions with, 64
  web resources on, 65
Ataxic movement, in cerebral palsy, 97

Athetoid movement, in cerebral palsy,
    97
Atlantoaxial instability (AAI), in Down
    syndrome, 147
Atrial septal defect, 119
Atrioventricular canal defect, 119
Attention deficit/hyperactivity disorder
    (ADHD),
  assessment tools for, 69
  body functions and structures
    affected by, 69
  case example of, 70b
  diagnostic criteria for, 67
  epidemiology of, 67
  etiology of, 67
  evaluation of, 69
  interventions for, 70b
  performance skills affected by, 68
  precautions with, 69
  subtypes of, 67
  web resources on, 71
Auditory processing disorders, 207
Autism spectrum disorder(s) (ASDs),
  areas of occupation affected by, 76
  Asperger's syndrome as, 74
  assessment tools for, 77
  autistic disorder as, 73
  body functions and structures
    affected by, 77
  case example of, 79b
  childhood disintegrative disorder as,
    75
  classification of, 73
  epidemiology of, 73
  evaluation of, 77
  interventions for, 78b
  performance patterns affected by,
    76
  performance skills affected by, 76
  pervasive developmental disorder–
    not otherwise specified as, 74
  precautions with, 77
  Rett's syndrome as, 75
  web resources on, 79
Autistic disorder, 73

B

BADS (Behavioral Assessment of the
    Dysexecutive Syndrome), 373
Balcones Sensory Integration Screening
    Kit (BSI), 372
BASC (Behavioral Assessment System
    for Children), 373
Bay Area Functional Performance
    Evaluation (BaFPE), 372

Bayley Scale of Infant Development (BSID), 372

Beery-Buktenica Developmental Test of Visual-Motor Integration (VMI), 372

Behavioral Assessment of the Dysexecutive Syndrome (BADS), 373

Behavioral Assessment System for Children (BASC), 373

Benton Constructional Praxis Test, 373

Bipolar disorder,
   assessment tools for, 83
   body functions and structures affected by, 82
   case example of, 84b
   clinical features of, 81
   epidemiology of, 81
   evaluation of, 83
   interventions for, 84b
   performance skills affected by, 81
   precautions with, 83
   web resources on, 84

Bleeding episodes, in hemophilia, 175

BOT-2 (Bruininks-Oseretsky Test of Motor Performance), 373

Box and Block test, 373

BPD. *See* Bronchopulmonary dysplasia (BPD).

Brachial plexus injury,
   assessment tools for, 87
   body functions and structures affected by, 86
   case example of, 88b
   clinical features of, 86f
   epidemiology of, 85
   etiology of, 85
   evaluation of, 87
   interventions for, 87b
   performance skills affected by, 85
   precautions with, 86
   types of, 85
   web resources on, 88

Brachial plexus palsy. *See* Brachial plexus injury.

Bracing, for scoliosis, 323

Brain injury, acquired. *See* Acquired brain injury (ABI).

Breast milk jaundice, 185

Brittle bone disease. *See* Osteogenesis imperfecta (OI).

Bronchopulmonary dysplasia (BPD),
   body functions and structures affected by, 90
   case example of, 90b

Bronchopulmonary dysplasia (BPD) *(Continued)*
   epidemiology of, 89
   etiology of, 89
   evaluation of, 90
   interventions for, 90b
   medical treatment of, 89
   occupational performance affected by, 89
   performance patterns affected by, 89
   precautions with, 90
   web resource on, 90

Bruininks-Oseretsky Test of Motor Performance (BOT-2), 373

BSI (Balcones Sensory Integration Screening Kit), 372

BSID (Bayley Scale of Infant Development), 372

Bulimia,
   areas of occupation affected by, 93
   assessment tools for, 94
   body functions and structures affected by, 94
   case example of, 95b
   clinical features of, 93
   epidemiology of, 93
   evaluation of, 94
   interventions for, 95b
   performance skills affected by, 93
   precautions with, 94
   web resources on, 95

"Burners." *See* Brachial plexus injury.

C

Canadian Occupational Performance Measure (COPM), 374

CanChild Centre for Disability Research website, 367

CAPE (Children's Assessment of Participation and Enjoyment), 374

Carrier, of Tay-Sachs disease, 355

Cataracts, in galactosemia, 169, 170f

CBCL (Child Behavior Checklist), 374

CBI (Child Behaviors Inventory of Playfulness), 374

Centers for Disease Control and Prevention website, 368

Cerebral palsy (CP),
   assessment tools for, 105
   ataxic, 97
   athetoid, 97
   body functions and structures affected by, 99b
   case example of, 106b

Cerebral palsy (CP) *(Continued)*
classification of, 97, 99t, 100t
clinical features of, 97, 98f
diplegia in, 97
epidemiology of, 97
evaluation of, 105
hemiplegia in, 97
hypotonic, 97
interventions for, 106b
mixed, 97
performance skills affected by, 98
precautions with, 105
quadriplegia in, 97
spastic, 97
web resources on, 106
CF. *See* Cystic fibrosis (CF).
Cherry-red spot, in macula, 356f
CHES (Children's Handwriting
Evaluation Scale), 375
Child and Adolescent Social Perception
Measure, 374
Child Behavior Checklist (CBCL), 374
Child Behaviors Inventory of
Playfulness (CBI), 374
Child Occupational Self Assessment
(COSA), 374
Childhood disintegrative disorder, 75
Children's Assessment of Participation
and Enjoyment (CAPE), 374
Children's Handwriting Evaluation
Scale (CHES), 375
Children's Paced Auditory Serial
Addition Test (CHIPASAT),
375
Choosing Outcomes and
Accommodations for Children
(COACH), 375
Classroom Observation Guide, 375
Cleft palate,
body functions and structures
affected by, 107
case example of, 109b
clinical features of, 108f
epidemiology of, 107
etiology of, 107
evaluation of, 108
interventions for, 109b
medical treatment of, 107
occupational participation affected
by, 107
performance skills affected by, 107
precautions with, 108
web resources on, 109
Clinical question, in evidence-based
practice, 9

Clubfoot,
assessment tools for, 116
body functions and structures
affected by, 116
case example of, 117b
clinical features of, 115, 116f
epidemiology of, 115
evaluation of, 116
interventions for, 117b
medical treatment of, 115
performance skills affected by, 115
precautions with, 116
web resource on, 117
COACH (Choosing Outcomes and
Accommodations for Children),
375
Coagulation, disseminated
intravascular. *See* Disseminated
intravascular coagulation
(DIC).
Coarctation of the aorta, 119
Cochrane Reviews website, 368
Collaborative process model, in
Occupational Therapy Practice
Framework, 7f, 8
Community colleges, search engines at,
11
Computer System Usability
Questionnaire, 375
Conduct disorder,
assessment tools for, 112
body functions and structures
affected by, 112
case example of, 113b
clinical features of, 111
epidemiology of, 111
evaluation of, 112
interventions for, 113b
occupational performance affected
by, 111
performance patterns affected by, 112
performance skills affected by, 112
precautions with, 112
web resources on, 113
Congenital clubfoot. *See* Clubfoot.
Congenital heart defects. *See* Heart
defects, congenital.
Congenital obstructive hydrocephalus.
See Hydrocephalus, congenital
obstructive.
Continuing education courses,
gathering evidence from, 12
Coping Inventory, 375
COPM (Canadian Occupational
Performance Measure), 374

COSA (Child Occupational Self
  Assessment), 374
CP. *See* Cerebral palsy (CP).
Cri du chat syndrome,
  assessment tools for, 128
  body functions and structures
    affected by, 128
  case example of, 129b
  clinical features of, 127
  epidemiology of, 127
  etiology of, 127
  evaluation of, 128
  interventions for, 128b
  performance skills affected by, 127
  precautions with, 128
  web resources on, 129
Cystic fibrosis (CF),
  assessment tools for, 132
  body functions and structures
    affected by, 131
  case example of, 132b
  clinical features of, 131
  epidemiology of, 131
  evaluation of, 132
  interventions for, 132b
  performance patterns affected by,
    131
  performance skills affected by, 131
  precautions with, 132
  web resources on, 133

D

DCD. *See* Developmental coordination
  disorder (DCD).
DDAVP (desmopressin acetate), for
  hemophilia, 176
DeGangi-Berk Test of Sensory
  Integration (TSI), 376
Denver Developmental Screening Test
  (DDST), 376
Depression,
  assessment tools for, 137
  body functions and structures
    affected by, 136
  case example of, 138b
  epidemiology of, 135
  etiology of, 135
  evaluation of, 137
  interventions for, 138b
  performance skills affected by, 135
  precautions with, 137
  signs and symptoms of, 135
  web resources on, 138
Desmopressin acetate (DDAVP), for
  hemophilia, 176

Developmental coordination disorder
  (DCD),
  assessment tools for, 140
  body functions and structures
    affected by, 139
  case example of, 141b
  epidemiology of, 139
  evaluation of, 140
  interventions for, 141b
  performance skills affected by, 139
  precautions with, 139
  symptoms of, 139
  web resources on, 141
Developmental Test of Visual
  Perception (DTVP), 376
Diabetes
  defined, 199
  juvenile,
    body functions and structures
      affected by, 200
    epidemiology of, 199
    etiology of, 199
    medical treatment of, 199
    performance patterns affected by,
      200
    precautions with, 200
    signs and symptoms of, 199
    web resources on, 200
  types of, 199
Diplegia, in cerebral palsy, 97
Discussion boards, gathering evidence
  from, 12
Disseminated intravascular coagulation
  (DIC),
  assessment tools for, 144
  body functions and structures
    affected by, 143
  epidemiology of, 143
  etiology of, 143
  evaluation of, 144
  interventions for, 144b
  performance skills affected by, 143
  precautions with, 144
  signs and symptoms of, 143
  web resource on, 144
DOTCA-Ch (Dynamic Occupational
  Therapy Cognitive Assessment
  for Children), 376
Down syndrome (DS),
  assessment tools for, 148
  atlantoaxial instability in, 147
  body functions and structures
    affected by, 147
  case example of, 149b
  clinical features of, 145, 146f

Down syndrome (DS) *(Continued)*
  epidemiology of, 145
  etiology of, 145
  evaluation of, 148
  interventions for, 149b
  performance skills affected by, 147
  precautions with, 147
  web resources on, 149
DTVP (Developmental Test of Visual
      Perception), 376
Duchenne muscular dystrophy, 241,
      242f
Ductus arteriosus, patent, 119
Dwarfism. *See* Achondroplasia.
Dynamic Occupational Therapy
      Cognitive Assessment for
      Children (DOTCA-Ch), 376
Dyscalculia, 207
Dysgraphia, 207
Dyslexia, 207
Dysrhythmias,
  assessment tools for, 152
  body functions and structures
      affected by, 151
  clinical features of, 151
  epidemiology of, 151
  etiology of, 151
  evaluation of, 152
  intervention for, 152b
  performance skills affected by, 151
  precautions with, 152
  web resources on, 152
Dystrophinopathies, 241

E

Early Coping Inventory, 376
EDPA (Erhardt Developmental
      Prehension Assessment), 376
EDVA (Erhardt Developmental
      Vision Assessment, Revised),
      377
Edwards' syndrome,
  body functions and structures
      affected by, 155
  case example of, 155b
  clinical features of, 153, 154f
  epidemiology of, 153
  etiology of, 153
  evaluation of, 155
  interventions for, 155b
  performance skills affected by, 154
  precautions with, 155
  web resources on, 156
Electronic databases, 11
Empyemata, due to pneumonia, 304

Encephalopathy, hypoxic-ischemic. *See*
      Hypoxic-ischemic
      encephalopathy (HIE).
Enterocolitis, necrotizing. *See*
      Necrotizing enterocolitis.
Epilepsy,
  body functions and structures
      affected by, 158
  clinical features of, 157
  epidemiology of, 157
  evaluation of, 158
  intervention for, 158b
  performance skills affected by, 157
  precautions with, 158
  risk factors for, 157
  web resources on, 158
Erb-Duchenne palsy. *See* Brachial
      plexus injury.
Erb's palsy. *See* Brachial plexus injury.
Erhardt Developmental Prehension
      Assessment (EDPA), 376
Erhardt Developmental Vision
      Assessment, Revised (EDVA),
      377
Evaluation, in Occupational Therapy
      Practice Framework, 4, 6b
Evaluation Tool of Children's
      Handwriting (ETCH), 377
Evidence
  hierarchy of levels of, 13, 13t
  uncovering best, 10
Evidence-based practice, 9
  evaluating information and
      determining how to apply it in,
      12
  forming question in, 9
  hierarchy of levels of evidence in, 13,
      13t
  search engines in, 10, 11, 12
  uncovering best evidence in, 10
  websites in, 12
Experience of Leisure Scale, The
      (TELS), 377

F

Facioscapulohumeral muscular
      dystrophy, 242
Fetal alcohol effects (FAE), 161
Fetal alcohol syndrome disorders
      (FASDs),
  assessment tools for, 163
  body functions and structures
      affected by, 163
  case example of, 164b
  clinical features of, 161, 162f

Fetal alcohol syndrome disorders
(FASDs) *(Continued)*
  epidemiology of, 161
  evaluation of, 163
  interventions for, 164b
  performance skills affected by, 162
  precautions with, 163
  types of, 161
  web resources on, 164
Fetal circulation, persistent. *See*
    Persistent pulmonary
    hypertension of the newborn
    (PPHN).
Fibrillin-1, in Marfan syndrome, 225
Fine Motor Task Assessment, 377
FirstSTEp Developmental Screening
    Test, 377
Fragile X syndrome (FXS),
  assessment tools for, 167
  body functions and structures
    affected by, 166
  case example of, 168b
  clinical features of, 165, 166f
  diagnosis of, 165
  epidemiology of, 165
  etiology of, 165
  evaluation of, 167
  interventions for, 168b
  performance skills affected by, 165
  precautions with, 166
  web resources on, 168
Functional Independence Measure for
    Children (WeeFIM), 377
FXS. *See* Fragile X syndrome (FXS).

G

GAD (generalized anxiety disorder), 49
Galactosemia,
  assessment tools for, 171
  body functions and structures
    affected by, 170
  case example of, 172b
  cataracts in, 169, 170f
  clinical features of, 169, 170f
  epidemiology of, 169
  etiology of, 169
  evaluation of, 171
  interventions for, 172b
  performance skills affected by, 169
  precautions with, 170
  web resource on, 172
Gangliosides, in Tay-Sachs disease, 355
Gastroschisis,
  body functions and structures
    affected by, 173

Gastroschisis *(Continued)*
  case example of, 174b
  clinical features of, 174b
  epidemiology of, 173
  evaluation of, 174
  interventions for, 174b
  medical treatment of, 173
  occupational participation affected
    by, 173
  precautions with, 173
Generalized anxiety disorder (GAD),
    49
Google Scholar website, 368
Great arteries, transposition of, 119
Gross Motor Function Classification
    System (GMFCS), 98, 100t
Gross Motor Function Measure
    (GMFM), 377

H

Hawaii Early Learning Profile (HELP),
    377
Heart defects, congenital,
  assessment tools for, 121
  body functions and structures
    affected by, 121
  case example of, 122b
  epidemiology of, 119
  etiology of, 119
  evaluation of, 121
  interventions for, 122b
  medical treatment of, 119
  occupational performance affected
    by, 120
  performance patterns affected by,
    121
  performance skills affected by, 121
  precautions with, 121
  signs and symptoms of, 120
  types of, 119
  web resources on, 122
Heart rates, abnormal. *See*
    Dysrhythmias.
HELP (Hawaii Early Learning Profile),
    377
Hemiplegia, in cerebral palsy, 97
Hemolysis, jaundice from, 185
Hemophilia,
  assessment tools for, 176
  bleeding episodes in, 175
  body functions and structures
    affected by, 176
  case example of, 177b
  DDAVP for, 176
  defined, 175

Hemophilia (*Continued*)
  epidemiology of, 175
  etiology of, 175
  evaluation of, 176
  interventions for, 177b
  mild, 175
  moderate, 175
  performance skills affected by, 176
  precautions with, 176
  severe, 175
  signs and symptoms of, 175
  types of, 175
  web resources on, 177
Hemorrhage, intraventricular. See
    Intraventricular hemorrhage
    (IVH).
Hexosaminidase A, in Tay-Sachs
    disease, 355
HIE. See Hypoxic-ischemic
    encephalopathy (HIE).
Hip, ischemic necrosis of. See Legg-
    Calvé-Perthes disease.
HIV (human immunodeficiency virus).
    See Acquired immunodeficiency
    syndrome (AIDS).
Holoprosencephaly, in Patau's
    syndrome, 279
Home Observation and Measurement
    of the Environment (HOME),
    378
Horner's syndrome. See Brachial plexus
    injury.
HPRT (hypoxanthine-guanine
    phosphoriboxyltransferase), in
    Lesch-Nyhan syndrome, 217
Human immunodeficiency virus
    (HIV). See Acquired
    immunodeficiency syndrome
    (AIDS).
Hydrocephalus,
  acquired, 179
  assessment tools for, 182
  body functions and structures
    affected by, 181
  communicating, 179
  congenital obstructive,
    assessment tools for, 124
    body functions and structures
      affected by, 124
    case example of, 125b
    clinical features of, 123
    vs. communicating, 179
    epidemiology of, 123
    etiology of, 123

Hydrocephalus (*Continued*)
    evaluation of, 124
    interventions for, 125b
    medical treatment of, 123
    performance skills affected by, 123
    precautions with, 124
    web resources on, 125
  epidemiology of, 179
  etiology of, 179, 180f
  evaluation of, 181
  interventions for, 182b
  intraventricular shunts for, 181
  medical treatment of, 180f
  performance skills affected by, 179
  precautions with, 181
  web resource on, 183
Hyperactivity. See Attention deficit/
    hyperactivity disorder
    (ADHD).
Hyperbilirubinemia,
  body functions and structures
    affected by, 186
  defined, 185
  epidemiology of, 185
  etiology of, 185
  evaluation of, 186
  intervention for, 186b
  medical treatment of, 185
  precautions with, 186
  symptoms of, 185
  web resource on, 186
Hypertension, persistent pulmonary.
    See Persistent pulmonary
    hypertension of the newborn
    (PPHN).
Hypoplastic left heart syndrome, 119
Hypotonic movement, in cerebral
    palsy, 97
Hypoxanthine-guanine
    phosphoriboxyltransferase
    (HPRT), in Lesch-Nyhan
    syndrome, 217
Hypoxic-ischemic encephalopathy
    (HIE),
  assessment tools for, 188
  body functions and structures
    affected by, 188
  epidemiology of, 187
  etiology of, 187
  evaluation of, 188
  intervention for, 188b
  performance skills affected by, 188
  precautions with, 188
  signs of, 187
  web resource for, 188

I

IDs. *See* Intellectual disabilities (IDs).
Infant/Toddler Sensory Profile, 378
Infection(s)
    liver, jaundice from, 185
    opportunistic, with AIDS, 26
Intellectual disabilities (IDs),
    assessment tools for, 192
    body functions and structures
        affected by, 192
    case example of, 193b
    diagnostic criteria for, 191
    epidemiology of, 191
    etiology of, 191
    evaluation of, 192
    interventions for, 193b
    performance skills affected by, 191
    precautions with, 192
    web resources on, 193
Interest Checklist, 378
Intervention, in Occupational
        Therapy Practice Framework, 4,
        6b
Intervention implementation, 6
Intervention plan, 6
Intervention review, 6
Intraventricular hemorrhage (IVH),
    assessment tools for, 196
    body functions and structures
        affected by, 196
    case example of, 196b
    defined, 195
    epidemiology of, 195
    etiology of, 195
    evaluation of, 196
    grading of bleeds related to, 195
    intervention for, 196b
    long-term effects of, 196
    performance skills affected by, 196
    precautions with, 196
    symptoms of, 195
    web resources on, 197
Intraventricular shunts, 181
Ischemic necrosis of the hip. *See* Legg-
        Calvé-Perthes disease.
IVH. *See* Intraventricular hemorrhage
        (IVH).

J

Jaundice. *See also* Hyperbilirubinemia.
    breast milk, 185
    from hemolysis, 185
    from liver malfunction or infection,
        185
    physiologic, 185

Juvenile diabetes. *See* Diabetes,
        juvenile.
Juvenile rheumatoid arthritis (JRA),
    assessment tools for, 203
    body functions and structures
        affected by, 202
    case example of, 203b
    epidemiology of, 201
    evaluation of, 203
    interventions for, 203b
    pauciarticular, 201
    performance skills affected by, 201
    polyarticular, 201
    precautions with, 202
    signs and symptoms of, 201
    systemic, 201
    types of, 201
    web resources on, 204

K

Keywords, for gathering evidence, 12
Klein-Bell Activities of Daily Living
        Scale, 378
Klinefelter's syndrome,
    assessment tools for, 206
    body functions and structures
        affected by, 205
    case example of, 206b
    clinical features of, 205
    defined, 205
    epidemiology of, 205
    evaluation of, 205
    intervention for, 206b
    performance skills affected by, 205
    precautions with, 205
    web resources on, 206
Klumpke's palsy. *See* Brachial plexus
        injury.
Knox Cube Test, 378
Knox Preschool Play Scale, 378

L

Landouzy-Dejerine disease, 242
Lazy eye. *See* Amblyopia.
LBS (Leisure Boredom Scale), 378
Learning disabilities,
    assessment tools for, 210
    body functions and structures
        affected by, 209
    case example of, 211b
    defined, 207
    epidemiology of, 207
    evaluation of, 210
    interventions for, 211b
    performance skills affected by, 208

Learning disabilities *(Continued)*
  precautions with, 209
  symptoms of, 208
  types of, 207
  web resources on, 211
Legg-Calvé-Perthes disease,
  assessment tools for, 214
  body functions and structures
      affected by, 213
  case example of, 214b
  defined, 213
  epidemiology of, 213
  evaluation of, 214
  interventions for, 214b
  medical treatment of, 213
  performance skills affected by, 213
  precautions with, 214
  signs and symptoms of, 213
  web resources on, 215
Leisure Boredom Scale (LBS), 378
Leisure Competence Measure, 379
Leisure Diagnostic Battery, 379
Leisure Satisfaction Scale, 379
Lesch-Nyhan syndrome,
  assessment tools for, 218
  body functions and structures
      affected by, 218
  case example of, 219b
  clinical features of, 217
  epidemiology of, 217
  etiology of, 217
  evaluation of, 218
  interventions for, 219b
  performance skills affected by, 217
  precautions with, 218
  web resource on, 220
Leukomalacia, periventricular. *See*
      Periventricular leukomalacia
      (PVL).
Libraries, search engines at, 11
Lincoln-Oseretsky Motor Development
      Scale, 379
Liver infection, jaundice from, 185
Liver malfunction, jaundice from, 185
Lordosis,
  assessment tools for, 223
  body functions and structures
      affected by, 221
  case example of, 223b
  defined, 221, 222f
  epidemiology of, 221
  etiology of, 221
  evaluation of, 222
  interventions for, 223b
  medical treatment of, 221

Lordosis *(Continued)*
  performance skills affected by, 221
  precautions with, 222
  web resources on, 223
Lowenstein Occupational Therapy
      Cognitive Assessment (LOTCA),
      379
Lung abscesses, due to pneumonia,
      304

M

Macula, cherry-red spot in, 356f
MAI (Movement Assessment for
      Infants), 380
Manual Ability Classification System
      (MACS), 98, 99t
MAP (Miller Assessment for
      Preschoolers), 380
Marble-bone disease. *See* Albers-
      Schönberg disease.
Marfan syndrome,
  assessment tools for, 227
  body functions and structures
      affected by, 226, 227
  case example of, 227b
  clinical appearance of, 226f
  defined, 225
  epidemiology of, 225
  etiology of, 225
  evaluation of, 227
  intervention for, 227b
  performance skills affected by, 225,
      227
  precautions with, 227
  web resource on, 228
Mayo-Portland Adaptability Inventory
      (MPAI), 379
McCarthy Scale of Children's Abilities,
      379
MD. *See* Muscular dystrophy (MD).
Meconium, defined, 229
Meconium aspiration syndrome,
  assessment tools for, 231
  body functions and structures
      affected by, 230, 231
  case example of, 232b
  clinical features of, 229, 230f
  epidemiology of, 229
  etiology of, 229
  evaluation of, 231
  interventions for, 231b
  performance skills affected by, 229,
      230
  precautions with, 230
  web resource on, 232

M-FUN-S (Miller Function and
    Participation Scales), 380
Micrognathia,
  assessment tools for, 235
  body functions and structures
    affected by, 233, 235
  case example of, 235b
  clinical features of, 234f
  defined, 233
  epidemiology of, 233
  evaluation of, 235
  interventions for, 235b
  performance skills affected by, 233,
    234
  precautions with, 234
  web resource on, 236
Miller Assessment for Preschoolers
  (MAP), 380
Miller Function and Participation
  Scales (M-FUN-S), 380
Mixed movement disorder, in cerebral
  palsy, 97
Model of Human Occupation
  (MOHO) Clearinghouse
  website, 368
Model of Human Occupation
  Screening Tool (MOHOST),
  380
Mononucleosis,
  assessment tools for, 238
  body functions and structures
    affected by, 238
  case example of, 239b
  clinical features of, 237
  defined, 237
  epidemiology of, 237
  etiology of, 237
  evaluation of, 238
  interventions for, 239b
  performance skills affected by, 237,
    238
  precautions with, 238
  web resource on, 239
Mother-Child Interaction Checklist,
  380
Motor Assessment Battery for Children
  (Movement ABC), 380
Movement Assessment for Infants
  (MAI), 380
MPAI (Mayo-Portland Adaptability
  Inventory), 379
Muscular dystrophy (MD),
  assessment tools for, 244
  body functions and structures
    affected by, 243, 244

Muscular dystrophy (MD) *(Continued)*
  case example of, 245b
  clinical features of, 241, 242f
  defined, 241
  Duchenne, 241, 242f
  dystrophinopathies, 241
  epidemiology of, 241
  evaluation of, 244
  facioscapulohumeral, 242
  interventions for, 245b
  myotonic, 242
  performance skills affected by, 243,
    244
  precautions with, 244
  web resource on, 245
Myotonic dystrophy, 242

N

National Institutes of Health (NIH)
  Activity Record, 381
National Institutes of Health (NIH)
  website, 11, 368
Necrotizing enterocolitis,
  assessment tools for, 249
  body functions and structures
    affected by, 248
  case example of, 249b
  defined, 247
  epidemiology of, 247
  etiology of, 247
  evaluation of, 249
  interventions for, 249b
  performance skills affected by, 247,
    248
  precautions with, 248
  risk factors for, 247
  web resources on, 250
Neonatal respiratory distress
  syndrome,
  assessment tools for, 253
  body functions and structures
    affected by, 252
  case example of, 254b
  epidemiology of, 251
  etiology of, 251
  evaluation of, 253
  interventions for, 253b
  performance skills affected by, 251,
    252
  precautions with, 252
  web resource on, 254
Neurofibromatosis type 1 (NF-1),
  assessment tools for, 257
  body functions and structures
    affected by, 256, 257

Neurofibromatosis type 1 (NF-1)
    (Continued)
  case example of, 258b
  clinical features of, 255, 256, 257
  defined, 255
  epidemiology of, 255
  evaluation of, 257
  interventions for, 258b
  performance skills affected by, 255,
    256
  precautions with, 256
  web resources on, 258
Neurofibromatosis type 2 (NF-2), 256
NIH (National Institutes of Health)
    Activity Record, 381
NIH (National Institutes of Health)
    website, 11, 368
Nowicki-Strickland Locus of Control
    Scale for Children [TIM(C)],
    381
Nystagmus,
  acquired, 261, 262
  assessment tools for, 263
  body functions and structures
    affected by, 262
  case example of, 263b
  congenital, 261, 262
  defined, 261
  epidemiology of, 261
  evaluation of, 263
  grading of, 262
  interventions for, 263b
  performance skills affected by,
    262
  precautions with, 262
  spasmus nutans, 261
  web resources on, 263

O

Obesity,
  assessment tools for, 266
  body functions and structures
    affected by, 265, 266
  case example of, 267b
  defined, 265
  epidemiology of, 265
  evaluation of, 266
  interventions for, 266b
  vs. overweight, 265
  performance skills affected by, 265,
    266
  due to Prader-Willi syndrome, 307,
    309, 308f
  precautions with, 266
  web resource on, 267

Obstructive hydrocephalus, congenital.
    See Hydrocephalus, congenital
    obstructive.
Occupational Circumstances
    Assessment Interview and
    Rating Scale (OCAIRS), 381
Occupational performance, analysis of,
    6
Occupational Performance History
    Interview (OPHI), 381
Occupational profile, 6
Occupational therapy
  creation of unified language for, 3
  domain of, 4, 5f
Occupational Therapy Critically
    Appraised Topics website, 369
Occupational Therapy Practice
    Framework, 4
  domains in, 4, 5f
  evaluation in, 4, 6b
  intervention in, 4, 6b
  outcomes in, 4, 6b
  overview of, 7f, 8
  service delivery in, 4, 6b
OI. *See* Osteogenesis imperfecta (OI).
OPHI (Occupational Performance
    History Interview), 381
Opportunistic infections, with AIDS, 26
Oppositional defiant disorder (ODD),
  assessment tools for, 271
  body functions and structures
    affected by, 270
  case example of, 271b
  epidemiology of, 269
  evaluation of, 270
  interventions for, 271b
  performance skills affected by, 269,
    270
  precautions with, 270
  signs and symptoms of, 269
  web resources on, 271
Osteogenesis imperfecta (OI),
  assessment tools for, 275
  body functions and structures
    affected by, 273, 274
  case example of, 276b
  clinical features of, 274f
  epidemiology of, 273
  etiology of, 273
  evaluation of, 275
  interventions for, 275b
  performance skills affected by, 273,
    274
  precautions with, 274
  web resource on, 276

Osteopetrosis. *See* Albers-Schönberg disease.
OT Seeker, 10, 369
OT-CATS, 11
Outcomes, in Occupational Therapy Practice Framework, 4, 6b

P

5p–syndrome. *See* Cri du chat syndrome.
PACS (Pediatric Activity Card Sort), 381
PACS (Preferences for Activities for Children), 382
Patau's syndrome,
    assessment tools for, 280
    body functions and structures affected by, 278, 279
    case example of, 280b
    clinical features of, 278f
    defined, 277
    epidemiology of, 277
    evaluation of, 280
    holoprosencephaly in, 279
    interventions for, 280b
    performance skills affected by, 277, 279
    precautions with, 279
    web resources on, 280
Patent ductus arteriosus, 119
PDD-NOS (pervasive developmental disorder–not otherwise specified), 74
Peabody Developmental Motor Scales 2 (PDMS-2), 381
Pediatric Activity Card Sort (PACS), 381
Pediatric Evaluation of Disability Inventory (PEDI), 382
Pediatric Interest Profile (PIP), 382
Pediatric Volitional Questionnaire (PVQ), 382
Perceived Efficacy and Goal Setting System (PEGS), 382
Periventricular leukomalacia (PVL),
    assessment tools for, 284
    body functions and structures affected by, 284
    case example of, 285b
    defined, 283
    epidemiology of, 283
    etiology of, 283
    evaluation of, 284

Periventricular leukomalacia (PVL) *(Continued)*
    interventions for, 285b
    performance skills affected by, 283, 284
    precautions with, 284
    web resource on, 285
Persistent fetal circulation. *See* Persistent pulmonary hypertension of the newborn (PPHN).
Persistent pulmonary hypertension of the newborn (PPHN),
    assessment tools for, 289
    body functions and structures affected by, 288
    case example of, 289b
    defined, 287
    epidemiology of, 287
    evaluation of, 289
    interventions for, 289b
    pathophysiology of, 287
    performance skills affected by, 287, 288
    precautions with, 288
    signs of, 288
    web resources on, 290
Pervasive developmental disorder–not otherwise specified (PDD-NOS), 74
Phenylketonuria (PKU),
    assessment tools for, 292
    body functions and structures affected by, 292
    case example of, 293b
    defined, 291
    epidemiology of, 291
    evaluation of, 292
    interventions for, 293b
    performance skills affected by, 291, 292
    precautions with, 292
    web resources on, 293
Phobia, social. *See* Social phobia.
Physiologic jaundice, 185
Pica,
    assessment tools for, 296
    body functions and structures affected by, 295, 296
    case example of, 297b
    complications of, 295, 296
    defined, 295
    epidemiology of, 295
    evaluation of, 296
    interventions for, 297b

Pica *(Continued)*
  performance skills affected by, 295, 296
  precautions with, 296
  web resources on, 297
PIP (Pediatric Interest Profile), 382
PKBS (Preschool and Kindergarten Behavior Scales), 383
PKU. *See* Phenylketonuria (PKU).
Pneumonia,
  assessment tools for, 305
  bacterial, 303
  body functions and structures affected by, 304
  case example of, 305b
  defined, 303
  empyemata due to, 304
  epidemiology of, 303
  etiology of, 303
  evaluation of, 305
  interventions for, 305b
  performance skills affected by, 303, 304
  precautions with, 304
  signs and symptoms of, 304
  viral, 303
  web resources on, 305
Posttraumatic stress disorder (PTSD),
  assessment tools for, 301
  body functions and structures affected by, 300
  case example of, 301b
  epidemiology of, 299
  etiology of, 299
  evaluation of, 300
  interventions for, 301b
  performance skills affected by, 299, 300
  precautions with, 300
  web resources on, 301
PPHN. *See* Persistent pulmonary hypertension of the newborn (PPHN).
Prader-Willi syndrome (PWS),
  assessment tools for, 310
  body functions and structures affected by, 309
  case example of, 310b
  clinical features of, 308f
  defined, 307
  epidemiology of, 307
  evaluation of, 309
  interventions for, 310b
  obesity due to, 307, 309

Prader-Willi syndrome (PWS) *(Continued)*
  performance skills affected by, 307, 309
  precautions with, 309
  signs of, 309
  web resources on, 310
Preferences for Activities for Children (PACS), 382
Prematurity, retinopathy of. *See* Retinopathy of prematurity (ROP).
Preschool and Kindergarten Behavior Scales (PKBS), 383
PTSD. *See* Posttraumatic stress disorder (PTSD).
PubMed, 11, 368
Pulmonary atresia, 119
Pulmonary hypertension, persistent. *See* Persistent pulmonary hypertension of the newborn (PPHN).
Pulmonary stenosis, 119
Pulmonary venous connection, total anomalous, 119
PVL. *See* Periventricular leukomalacia (PVL).
PVQ (Pediatric Volitional Questionnaire), 382
PWS. *See* Prader-Willi syndrome (PWS).

Q

Quadriplegia, in cerebral palsy, 97
Question, in evidence-based practice, 9

R

Respiratory distress syndrome, neonatal. *See* Neonatal respiratory distress syndrome.
Retinopathy of prematurity (ROP),
  assessment tools for, 315
  body functions and structures affected by, 315
  case example of, 316b
  clinical features of, 314f
  defined, 313
  epidemiology of, 313
  etiology of, 313
  evaluation of, 315
  interventions for, 316b
  performance skills affected by, 313, 315

Retinopathy of prematurity (ROP)
  (Continued)
  precautions with, 315
  web resources on, 316
Rett's syndrome, 75
Rheumatic fever, 317
Rheumatic heart disease,
  assessment tools for, 319
  body functions and structures
    affected by, 318
  case example of, 319b
  epidemiology of, 317
  etiology of, 317
  evaluation of, 318
  interventions for, 319b
  performance skills affected by, 317,
    318
  precautions with, 318
  symptoms of, 318
  treatment of, 317
  web resource on, 319
Rheumatoid arthritis, juvenile. *See*
    Juvenile rheumatoid arthritis
    (JRA).
ROP. *See* Retinopathy of prematurity
    (ROP).

S

SAOF (Self-Assessment of
    Occupational Functioning),
    383
School Assessment of Motor and
    Process Skills (School AMPA),
    383
School Function Assessment (SFA), 383
School Sensory Profile, 383
School Setting Interview (SSI), 383
Scoliosis,
  assessment tools for, 324
  body functions and structures
    affected by, 322, 323
  bracing for, 323
  case example of, 325b
  congenital, 321, 324
  defined, 321, 322f
  epidemiology of, 321
  etiology of, 321
  evaluation of, 324
  idiopathic, 321, 323
  interventions for, 324b
  neuromuscular, 321, 324
  performance skills affected by, 321,
    323
  precautions with, 323
  web resources on, 325

SCOPE (Short Child Occupational
    Profile), 384
Search engines
  occupational therapy, 10
  other scholarly, 11
  popular, 12
Seizure(s)
  defined, 157
  warning signs of, 158
Seizure disorder. *See* Epilepsy.
Self-Assessment of Occupational
    Functioning (SAOF), 383
Sensory processing, defined, 331
Sensory processing disorder (SPD),
  assessment tools for, 333
  body functions and structures
    affected by, 332, 333
  case example of, 334b
  epidemiology of, 331
  evaluation of, 333
  interventions for, 333b
  performance skills affected by, 331,
    332
  precautions with, 332
  web resources on, 334
Sensory Processing Measure (SPM),
    384
Sensory Profile, 384
Separation anxiety,
  assessment tools for, 329
  body functions and structures
    affected by, 328
  case example of, 329b
  epidemiology of, 327
  evaluation of, 328
  interventions for, 329b
  performance skills affected by, 327,
    328
  precautions with, 328
  web resources on, 329
Sepsis,
  assessment tools for, 336
  body functions and structures
    affected by, 336
  case example of, 337b
  defined, 335
  epidemiology of, 335
  evaluation of, 336
  interventions for, 337b
  performance skills affected by, 335,
    336
  precautions with, 336
  sequelae of, 336
  signs and symptoms of, 336
  web resources on, 337

Service delivery, in Occupational Therapy Practice Framework, 4, 6b

SFA (School Function Assessment), 383

Short Child Occupational Profile (SCOPE), 384

Shunt, for hydrocephalus, 180f

Sickle cell anemia,
  assessment tools for, 341
  body functions and structures affected by, 339, 340f, 341
  case example of, 341b
  defined, 339
  epidemiology of, 339
  evaluation of, 341
  interventions for, 341b
  performance skills affected by, 339, 341
  precautions with, 341
  web resources on, 342

SMA. *See* Spinal muscular atrophy (SMA).

Social phobia,
  assessment tools for, 329
  body functions and structures affected by, 328
  case example of, 329b
  epidemiology of, 327
  evaluation of, 328
  interventions for, 329b
  performance skills affected by, 327, 328
  precautions with, 328
  web resources on, 329

Social Skills Rating System, 384

Spasmus nutans, 261

Spastic movement, in cerebral palsy, 97

SPD. *See* Sensory processing disorder (SPD).

Spina bifida,
  assessment tools for, 345
  body functions and structures affected by, 344, 345
  case example of, 346b
  clinical features of, 344f
  epidemiology of, 343
  etiology of, 343
  evaluation of, 345
  interventions for, 346b
  performance skills affected by, 343, 344
  precautions with, 344
  web resources on, 346

Spinal muscular atrophy (SMA),
  assessment tools for, 348
  body functions and structures affected by, 348
  case example of, 349b
  epidemiology of, 347
  evaluation of, 348
  interventions for, 349b
  performance skills affected by, 347, 348
  precautions with, 348
  web resources on, 349

SPM (Sensory Processing Measure), 384

SSI (School Setting Interview), 383

Steinert's disease, 242

"Stingers." *See* Brachial plexus injury.

Strabismus,
  assessment tools for, 352
  body functions and structures affected by, 352
  case example of, 353b
  defined, 351
  epidemiology of, 351
  etiology of, 351
  evaluation of, 352
  interventions for, 353b
  performance skills affected by, 351, 352
  precautions with, 352
  web resources on, 353

Stress, posttraumatic. *See* Posttraumatic stress disorder (PTSD).

T

Talipes equinovarus. *See* Clubfoot.

Tay-Sachs disease,
  assessment tools for, 357
  body functions and structures affected by, 357
  carrier of, 355
  case example of, 358b
  clinical features of, 356f
  defined, 355
  epidemiology of, 355
  etiology of, 355
  evaluation of, 357
  interventions for, 358b
  performance skills affected by, 355, 357
  precautions with, 357
  web resources on, 358

TELS (The Experience of Leisure Scale), 377

Test of Environmental Supportiveness, 384

Test of Everyday Attention for Children (TEA-Ch), 384

Test of Sensory Integration (TSI), DeGangi-Berk, 376

Test of Visual-Motor Skills: Upper Level (TVMS:UL), 385

Test of Visual-Perceptual Skills (TVPS-3), 385

Test of Visual-Perceptual Skills: Upper Level (Non-Motor) (TVPS:UL), 385

Tetralogy of Fallot, 119

Tics, in Tourette syndrome, 361

TIM(C) (Nowicki-Strickland Locus of Control Scale for Children), 381

Toddler and Infant Motor Evaluation (TIME), 385

Total anomalous pulmonary venous connection, 119

Tourette syndrome,
  assessment tools for, 362
  body functions and structures affected by, 361, 362
  case example of, 362b
  epidemiology of, 361
  evaluation of, 362
  interventions for, 362b
  performance skills affected by, 361, 362
  precautions with, 362
  tics in, 361
  web resources on, 363

Transposition of the great arteries, 119

Trauma, posttraumatic stress disorder due to. *See* Posttraumatic stress disorder (PTSD).

Tricuspid atresia, 119

Trisomy 13. *See* Patau's syndrome.

Trisomy 18. *See* Edwards' syndrome.

Trisomy 21. *See* Down syndrome (DS).

Truncus arteriosus, 119

TSI (DeGangi-Berk Test of Sensory Integration), 376

TVMS:UL (Test of Visual-Motor Skills: Upper Level), 385

TVPS-3 (Test of Visual-Perceptual Skills), 385

TVPS:UL [Test of Visual-Perceptual Skills: Upper Level (Non-Motor)], 385

U

Uniform Terminology, 4

U.S. Library of National Medicine website, 369

V

Ventricular septal defect, 119

Vineland Adaptive Behavior Scale (VABS), 385

Visual processing disorders, 207

Visual-Motor Integration (VMI), Beery-Buktenica Developmental Test of, 372

von Recklinghausen's disease. *See* Neurofibromatosis type 1 (NF-1).

W

Web-based discussion boards, gathering evidence from, 12

Websites, for research, 12

WeeFIM (Functional Independence Measure for Children), 377

Wrightslaw Special Education Law and Advocacy website, 369